A Guide to *Transformation* and *Leadership* for a
Relationship-Centric Healthcare Culture

28 Ways of Compassion

DEE BORGOYN

RIVER GROVE
BOOKS

Dee Borgoyn ♡

Published by River Grove Books

Austin, TX
www.rivergrovebooks.com

Distributed by River Grove Books

Design and composition by Greenleaf Book Group
Cover design by Greenleaf Book Group and Chantel Stull
Cover image by ©Shutterstock.com/Cluckva

Publisher's Cataloging-in-Publication data is available.

Print ISBN: 978-1-63299-202-4

eBook ISBN: 978-1-63299-203-1

First Edition

This book is dedicated to my daughter Denae. She is the joy and the pride of my life. Her bravery, grace, and compassion are an inspiration to me and everyone around her. She is becoming a wonderful healthcare leader in her own right, as well as being an incredible wife, friend, and mother to my grand-daughter Tiana.

Denae, you are always and forever my hero!

Contents

Acknowledgments

Where to start to thank all the people who have encouraged and driven the writing of this book?!

First, I want to thank my husband, Kurt Borgoyn. He has been my rock for over fifteen years, and the unwavering supporter that kept me pushing and striving to get it done. He wholeheartedly believes in me and the passion I have for what I do. His unwavering acceptance of and faith in me keeps me going every day.

This book would not have been possible without the skills and confidence of some wonderful people at Greenleaf Book Group. When I saw Tanya Hall, CEO, speak at a conference I was drawn to approach her about this book proposal, because I felt like they were the publisher that would help me make this happen. Carolyn Roark was my first editor, tasked with partnering with me to produce a working manuscript. She truly had her work cut out for her. I did not make it easy. She is a great coach and a wealth of information. With perseverance and the right balance of push, pull, and patience from Carolyn, we got it done together. Jay Hodges and Heather Stettler took it through the fine tuning.

Chantel Stull created the cover after listening carefully to my goals and visions. April Murphy and Jen Glynn were responsible for total project management. Thanks also to Sam Alexander and the distribution and marketing teams. From the outset Sam has helped me to stay focused on the market and my target audience. The Greenleaf Book Group has my wholehearted gratitude and respect for their talents, skills, and knowledge. Thank you all for believing in this project.

Deep thanks to the colleagues who've provided advice and support along the way. This includes fellow members of the National Speakers Association, which propels me in my dream career—especially Jennifer Fitzpatrick, Valerie Grubb, Dr. Shirley Davis, Dianna Booher, Ron Culberson, Liz Fletcher-Brown, and resources too numerous to name. Thank you to coworkers and consumers of health care services that have encouraged me by confirming the need for this book.

Thank you to my granddaughter Tiana Boyer, who followed along with my progress and searched online for quotes and information about compassion.

Lastly, thank you to all the nurses, doctors, nursing assistants, healthcare leaders, and people in general who've given me encouragement and provided real-life examples of 28 ways of compassion.

Introduction

"Too often we underestimate the power of a touch, a smile, a kind word, a listening ear, an honest compliment, or the smallest act of caring, all of which have the potential to turn a life around."

—LEO F. BUSCAGLIA

For as long as I can remember, I've been a student of people and their behavior. Humans are a continual source of fascination for me. I'm always observing, wondering what makes them tick, asking the question why.

Other than simple DNA, I think several factors in my life influenced this endless curiosity. Some are personal, and some are professional.

For example, from my earliest days I've experienced people through the point of view of someone with a physical difference. I was born with one hand, and I have used a hook prosthesis since before I could sit up. Watching how people react to a disability—negatively and positively—has taught me a lot about acceptance, inclusion, and compassion.

I was also raised in a military family. We moved every year or two until I started high school. I was always a "new kid," adjusting and finding my place in strange environments.

My family was dysfunctional in ways that I won't go into, and I'm the oldest, a girl, with two younger brothers. I spent a lot of time alone.

My youngest brother had learning difficulties and was slow to begin speaking. I made it my place to understand and communicate on his behalf, acting as an interpreter of sorts.

I grew up introspective, introverted, and sensitive to the feelings and needs of others. Sometimes too shy to be a participant, I've watched people dynamics throughout my life.

In college, I majored in special education with a minor in psychology. Through volunteer work I had discovered an affinity for people with special needs, and I wanted to make a difference in their lives. As fate would have it, however, there were no openings for teachers when it came time for me to graduate. I found an opportunity with a state agency providing services to people with physical and mental disabilities, which led me to a medical social worker role in a skilled nursing home.

Since then, for almost four decades, I've worked in healthcare and human services, sometimes on the front lines and sometimes in administration. But I've always worked with people.

I was advised before walking into an early job interview, "No matter what you do, don't say you *love* working with people. Every single applicant has said that the reason they're the best person for this job is that they *love* working with people." I've learned why they said that. It's because working with people can be frustrating, exhausting, maddening, and unrewarding. In fact most people who work with people every day, if they're being honest, wouldn't say they *love* working with them. But they would say they love helping people, that they enjoy and are challenged by them, and they like learning about and getting to know and understand them. They would also say they want to make a difference in people's lives.

I've studied leaders—good ones and not-so-good ones. I've coached and counseled staff as they've grown within companies from entry-level positions to top executive roles. I've hired thousands of people, trained them, developed them, and also laid off or in some cases fired them. My job has required root cause analysis of issues and development of correction and improvement strategies. I've needed to understand why people do what they do. When things go wrong, at what point did they go wrong? How could the problems have been prevented? Where we have successes, what are the common threads, and what can be duplicated? Beyond meeting the requirements of job descriptions and required competency checks, what behaviors and qualities make for exceptional staff in any environment?

I remember in the year 2000, while working in human resources for a large health-care system, that I was struck with the following question: Why is it that some nurses are able to stay productive and compassionate for decades, while some are not and slowly burn out and fade away? That question has been consistently in my mind through the years since. As an avid reader and lifelong learner, I've devoured publications, attended conferences, pursued more education, obtained certifications, studied teachings from experts ranging from the philosopher Aristotle to the Vietnamese monk Thich Nhat Hahn, and explored neurosciences, psychology, and wellness journals.

Some of the most meaningful information has come through my own qualitative research—watching the interactions of people in daily life at work and all around me. I truly started focusing on compassion in action, asking myself, "What just happened there?" and, "Why?" Everywhere I went . . . work, trains, hospitals, meetings, sitting at cafes, I took page after page of notes. Finding patterns, repetitions. Reading more books, comparing points to my notes. Whittling down and down until I realized that I'd identified 28 distinct ways that people act effectively with compassion. I then devised a usable, organized method to share them with you, in groups of 7 with 4 common themes, to help you categorize and internalize them. This book represents all of that studying and research in what I hope is a neat, compact 28 days/28 ways habit-forming regimen of compassion. My goal is to change your life by helping you to understand and practice compassionate behaviors in your own life and feel first-hand the difference these new habits make in your relationships with everyone around you.

How to
Use this Book

For Each Individual:

This book can strengthen your personal commitment to practicing more compassion, fortifying your own inner resources against "compassion fatigue," and helping you make a difference.

- Read the introduction and first three sections.

- Read and practice one chapter per day.

- Carry the book with you throughout the twenty-eight days.

- Write notes as you go through your day or at the end of the day. Your insights will be extremely valuable in helping you recognize the effects of intentional and active compassion.

- When you get to the end of the book, start over.

For Work Team Leaders:

If your organization has started a formal compassion initiative, the plan should be clearly communicated.

Caring and effective leaders can use this book independently to improve communication within work groups and enhance service and interactions for staff and patients or residents.

- Distribute a copy of the book to each member of your work team.

- Read these chapters together during staff meetings: *The Challenge*, *What Is Compassion?*, *Why We Need to Be Compassionate?*, and *Why We Withhold Compassion*.

- Assign each exercise to work within your team schedule. Explain to staff that each day's reading should only take ten minutes or so and should be done on scheduled work time. Allow your team extra time to read and take notes on Fridays and Mondays. Discuss with your staff together and one-on-one.

- Put some time on your regular staff meeting agenda to discuss points within the book. Have open discussions.

- Encourage staff to take notes in the book and share examples at staff meetings of how using compassion made a difference in their day for the patient, resident, or coworker.

- Be sure to use the compassion ideas in your own workday and pay close attention to how they are affecting you, as a leader and in your relationships with staff.

- Celebrate the difference!

For Organizations and Senior Leadership Groups:

Being a caring organization begins with accountable and effective executives. Leader behavior defines the culture—you don't just belong to it. Remember stewardship. The board decides what the culture should be—the leader defines and carries that out.

Ask yourself:

- Does this organization want to publicly declare itself to be a compassionate organization? This decision is made at the advisory board and senior leadership level.

  Think words like "intentional" and "thoughtful." These are powerful, declarative words that will immediately set a tone, establish expectations, and call attention to the quality of the interactions taking place.

  If the answer to this question is yes, then you must probe further.

- Is the organization ready to explore and commit to a simple plan to bring its most senior leaders, mid-level managers, and direct care/front-line staff on board?

Each member of the board and senior leadership team should read the book, so they can act as models before any compassion initiative begins.

The Challenge

"People don't care how much you know
until they know how much you care."

—ATTRIBUTED TO THEODORE ROOSEVELT

The people who provide our health care face unique challenges in applying what they know. They strive to give the recipient the most intimate and personal of services at a high quality while facing the complexities of medical practice management: extremely high financial overhead and risk and (for the foreseeable future) an unprecedented demand for services coupled with an insufficient and unreliable supply of people to provide them. With the aging population currently growing at a phenomenal rate, sometimes referred to as the gray tsunami, no discipline of the health-care industry is left unaffected. The truth is that the aging wave impacts every industry from housing to dining in some way, but it is health care that is at the front lines, in the trenches.

The elder living and senior services groups, in particular, are scrambling to meet the demands at their doors. Simple demographics mean many more people living longer with more complex physical conditions, yet wanting to "age in place." The aging services industry has no choice but to find real answers, and find them now.

As health-care providers are developing operational plans, there seems be an abundance of strategies and tools available for them to consider. These options may restate the problems and offer programs designed to organize and streamline processes. Some of the tactics are complicated and push groups to work harder, work smarter, work cheaper, and provide better customer service in the process.

These resources may fail to dig deep enough. They may just scratch the surface of this caring field that is so undeniably tied to the complicated interplay between human beings and the human existence. The resources and programs take time to institute, yet they may not stand the test of time. Often they're merely adhesive strips, "flavors of the month," quick fixes that react to the symptoms but don't address the basic underlying issues—bad connections between good people.

What if there was a way to adapt our behaviors so that we could feel more fulfilled, with an enhanced sense of accomplishment, like we made a difference through our work each day? The bad news is that there is no one magic global remedy. The good news is that there *is* a major component in attracting, retaining, and maximizing the productivity of caregiving staff while empowering everyone to serve the patient in a caring, understanding, and manageable way. This powerful tool has been lying directly underneath our noses, unexamined, unidentified, and untapped.

A Solution

This mysterious, powerful tool, this solution to healthcare's deeply rooted basic challenge is compassion.

Like Dorothy, who needed ruby slippers to show her that everything she wanted was right at home, or the farmer who searched far and wide only to find acres of diamonds on his own land, we have overlooked a natural key to some of our hardest-to-solve puzzles: how to attract and recruit enough qualified staff, how to retain them and keep them highly engaged, and how to enhance communication through all levels of our organization's communication. But the biggest puzzle of all is how to balance all of this against dollars—we face an enormous number of elderly patients living with serious health conditions, and payment for the care of those patients is based on quality experiences and outcomes. We all have the capacity for compassion within us, and through it we can unlock solutions to many health-care dilemmas.

Any organization that truly cares about or for people must embrace conscious compassion as a defined, tangible subject deserving of top priority on the strategic agenda. Jane Dutton, Professor Emeritus of Business Administration and Psychology at the University of Michigan, said, "When an organization's capacity for compassion comes from the top, it can result in a kind of compassion contagion that sweeps the whole organization."

Cold, unfeeling workplaces take their toll in turnover and stop discretionary efforts in their tracks. Where affection is shown at work, it seems to happen most often between coworkers; it rarely comes from management. Staff will report that they are highly connected and satisfied with their teammates but not with their leaders. Some studies are starting to suggest that when companies create more scenarios for leaders and management to interact directly with employees in positive ways, a more friendly, compassionate environment is created.

There is a growing body of research showing that a compassionate environment can nurture a workforce that is emotionally and physically healthy and that this is an increasingly competitive advantage for businesses across the spectrum.

It's becoming clear that organizations willing to explore compassion's complexities—its hows and whys, nuances, and manifestations—can reap the rewards of its far-reaching and culture-changing effects. However, before compassion can become part of organizational culture, we need a common language. This book offers a definition. We'll discuss why we need compassion, how we are healthier and happier when we show our compassion, and that we are born to be compassionate. Yes! Compassion is a feeling, a desire, that we all innately have. The word "compassion" is passive, it is a noun. It is the verb, to *be* compassionate by *acting on* that desire, that creates the connection.

Growing scientific evidence shows as well that withholding compassion actually creates harm to the self as well as others, and that individuals reap benefits from actively showing compassion. We'll also examine some reasons that we hold back from showing compassion.

What Is Compassion?

"All change, even very large and powerful change,
begins when a few people start talking with one another
about something they care about."

—MARGARET WHEATLEY

From recruiting and marketing materials to customer and resident/patient satisfaction training and surveys, from employee handbooks to company mission and vision statements, from HIPAA privacy declarations to patient rights proclamations, "care" and "caring" are terms that you can't help but notice are being communicated in every setting of the healthcare environment. A large proportion of the people who enter the field of healthcare do so because they have a heightened sense of caring. Sometimes it's based on a profound personal experience that has compelled them to become directly involved.

When we start to explain the meaning of caring and defining service to customers ("patients" in our world), we often begin the conversation by describing specific behavioral examples such as showing respect, paying attention to detail, anticipating needs ahead of time, and remembering to smile and make eye contact. There is another much more intimate level to human interactions and connections when they occur in the context of medical care: intimacy that is both physical and emotional, especially if one is on the receiving end. Compassion is honest, genuine, intimate, trustworthy, brave, optimistic, competent, realistic, and strong.

If we can start our conversation by suggesting a common understanding of the nature of both caring and compassion, then together we can build on that to envision a true transformation of the way we deliver health care. The first point of understanding to recognize and agree upon is that caring is not enough. We need to go deeper; we must reach beyond caring to an action—showing compassion.

The bridge between caring and compassion is traversed when we invest ourselves more deeply in those behavioral examples we named above. It happens when we move beyond actions and consider the hows and the whys of those actions. Contrary to what you may hear in the world of business, it *is* personal.

The second point of understanding is that compassion is a critical component for positive, effective professional communications and relationships. The absence of compassion underlies the number one organizational issue that I have seen consistently reflected in satisfaction and engagement surveys across all industries, in training needs assessments for both leadership *and* staff, and by both consumers *and* employees. That issue, and an organization's greatest challenge, is communication. Communication is arguably the prime center for the business training and development industry, augmented by the coaching and counseling of organizations. Poor communication has derailed many technically competent leaders and companies.

But communication is not enough. True connection does not occur without compassion. Here is a formula I suggest, to depict this concept:

> COMMUNICATION + COMPASSION = CONNECTION

Compassion is a core component of effective leadership, interpersonal relationships, communication, and real connection. On the front lines of direct caregiving, it is crucial for the caregiver to realize the need for self-compassion in order to safeguard their ability to provide care and services over the long term. When compassion is experienced, there often will be a feeling of lightening and gratitude.

Compassion is an openness, a willingness to share a common space and time with another human being. It is being fully present as a person, seeing the other in totality, without judgments. It is reaching out to meet another person where they are so that there can be the beginning of a shared understanding, even if not agreement. Again, neither party should leave having experienced a sense of loss of self. Compassion is a happening that results in a truer connection and positive outcomes for *both* parties.

Consider that compassion is better and more easily demonstrated than it is defined. *Compassion* as a term is a combination of the root word *com*, which means "together or common," and the word *passion*, which means "feeling," "drive," or "emotion" (typically to a strong or intense degree). Most definitions of *compassion* articulate something to the effect of a "sympathetic pity, concern, or sorrow for the struggles and misfortunes of others." So talking about compassion is a process of describing what is seen and felt. It's similar to love in that you kind of know it when you see it, or you can know its existence by the effect or impact that it has on those involved. It's like water and wind: invisible except in its effect and hard to capture, but you can feel it.

Being compassionate doesn't require a lot of training or preparation, but it does require a willingness to be present. Basic awareness itself can make you more compassionate. Any reader who starts practicing the compassion examples in this book should be able to feel an immediate difference in the quality of their personal interactions.

That said, this equation has to be considered at the organizational level as well as the personal level. Recently, I discussed compassion with a CEO, who said to me, "I think this is a great conversation to have. Obviously I don't need to be involved with it, but I really think it would be important for my managers to hear." Hmm.

Remember: In this business, it is personal. For meaningful, measurable changes to occur, all parties need to be involved, aware, and committed. For an organization to be compassionate, all stakeholders must see compassion as universal and fundamental to the way business is done. It is hard to share what you don't have.

For an industry-changing paradigm shift to occur, compassion has to be an active part of discussion and intentional action from the boardroom to the bedside.

There is absolutely no limit to the number or types of actions that can be taken or ways that compassion can be manifested. As soon as you make one comprehensive list, someone will come forward with another example of compassion in action. That's because every interaction, every singular situation, presents undeniably unique, nonreplicable opportunities for a shared human experience.

Why We Need to Be Compassionate

"Compassion will no longer be seen as a spiritual luxury
for a contemplative few. Rather it will be viewed
as a social necessity for the entire human family."

—DUANE ELGIN

There are those who have long dismissed soft subjects and skills such as compassion as touchy-feely, something that has no place or benefit in the business world. But scientists are starting to map a deep biological basis for our psychological needs back to the roots of evolution. The physical responses to compassion include a slowing of the heart and the secretion of a bonding hormone similar to oxytocin. Specific regions of the brain actually light up, resulting in the human desire to approach and care for another being. We can see that it exists, and we've felt it. Now we'll talk about why compassion is such a critical component of our daily lives, both at home and in the workplace.

As humans we are programmed to connect and belong. These are key basic needs, and inside we all yearn for the need for connection to be satisfied whether we recognize it or not. We need to be seen and heard. The word *intimacy* can be described as meaning "into me, see." If we feel that we've been seen and heard, then we tend to feel acknowledged and understood. Even if there is disagreement, we will tend to trust that the other party is aware of our views and has taken them into consideration.

Babies who do not receive nurturing in the form of human connection fail to thrive, even if they're getting adequate nutrition, hydration, and physical care.

We are born compassionate. Watch small children. They are empathetic, sympathetic, and compassionate all at once. Before they grow an adult filter, they will engage each other from across a room, cry or laugh in response to an unfamiliar child's stimulus, and leap out of their seat to help one another.

Their connection, like an automatic bond, is a delight to see. It is without guise or agenda. It is reaching out to a kindred spirit.

At work, the happiest and most fulfilled people tend to have found a vocation in which their personal self and their work self are not in conflict with one another but are congruent and aligned. We need to be able to bring "ourselves" to work.

In healthcare, we strive to hire staff who demonstrate caring for other people. When appropriate and given a choice between experience vs. naturally caring, I would hire the interviewee who consistently demonstrated the strongest concern and desire to help others.

Why We Withhold Compassion

"Maybe one of you can enlighten me, but I just don't
understand why it is so hard to be kind to one another."

—PATRICIA POLACCO

Many rewards come from being compassionate in our human
relationships, and we're inherently programmed to be compassionate. We actually have to go against our very nature when we
don't reach out. There are negative consequences for this holding
back, for both the other person and for ourselves. Yet there are
still times when we refrain from extending a smile, a touch, or a
word that would connect us to another human being.

Why? The biggest barrier is fear:

· Fear of risk to the organization if the line between business
and personal is crossed

· Fear that offering assistance will reveal needs too great or
impossible to fill

· Fear of not knowing what to say

- Fear of appearing soft or a bleeding heart
- Fear of accusations of favoritism or unequal treatment
- Fear that there isn't enough time to be compassionate
- Fear that showing compassion will somehow diminish power or status
- Fear of feeling helpless and overwhelmed
- Fear that emotional openness may cloud judgment or cause others to question judgment
- Fear of being unable to handle emotions, good or bad, or that connecting with others will hurt too much

We must face fear honestly and head-on if we're going to provide quality health care and services for the millions of people aging over the next several decades.

Not showing compassion does not mean that we're not compassionate. It means that there is something stopping us from taking action, and we need to discover what it is. It takes more effort to hold back compassion that we feel than it does to experience and act on it.

Take, for example, what is a sad daily occurrence in any large city, passing by a homeless person on the street. Many people will walk on by, acting as if they are totally unaware of the human being near them. They avoid any form of contact, even eye contact, instead paying rapt attention to someone or something else, or even nothing. I admit that in my discomfort I've sometimes done the same thing. I find that after I've passed I've felt relief.

But if I'm honest with myself I also realize that there's a vague sense of regret, sadness, maybe even shame about a missed opportunity to ease in some way the pain of another person.

The impact on a person who needs but isn't being shown compassion is a destruction of self: self-worth, self-esteem, self-respect, self-love. Over time he will build a shield to separate himself from the pain. He may shut down or withdraw, or, at the most severe, strike out and blame the people who've made him feel that he doesn't belong. These people will sometimes join together as bullies to find a sense of belonging. Bullies don't act alone. This is also why people find common enemies.

Each time we hold back our instinctive humanity it chips away a tiny piece of our heart. And holding back can be in conflict with our moral principles. Letting it flow feels so much better and more natural. Again, it takes less energy and, in fact, builds positive energy.

It's a simple but not easy answer. The first impulse of what to do is usually the best, most meaningful action. The 28 ways of compassion described in this book are designed to help set the stage for compassionate behavior, help you recognize what's holding you back, and provide concrete steps to get you started on the right track.

What's in It for Leadership?

An often-heard acronym in leadership, customer service, and training is W.I.I.F.M.? The letters stand for "What's In It For

Me?"[1] It's purported to be the key to convincing people that what you have is what they want, and that what you have is going to fulfill their need or solve a problem. Throughout this book you may notice explanations of how acting with compassion will benefit you; those explanations detail what's in it for you. But the deeper, non-selfish question is, "Why does compassion matter?" Or, more specific to this section, "Why does compassion matter in leadership?"

One of the primary jobs of leadership is to listen, understand, respect, and support their teams in the challenging work they do every day on the front lines.

Conscious compassion is central to leaders knowing their teams, and it drives the high level of staff engagement that results in happy, well-cared-for patients and residents. We are naturally compassionate, but we may not naturally know how to show it, especially at work and as a leader.

Leadership and service are founded on relationships. Relationships do not happen in an instant; they are built and grow stronger over time through repeated actions and habits as we foster understanding and trust. When we forge strong positive relationships on a consistent basis through positive, caring exchanges, it enables us to deal in a more productive way when the tough conversations and situations arise. While we won't necessarily have reached agreement, we may have come to respect and nurture a level of authenticity and the gift of confidence in

---

1 Or as my husband says, "Why am I wasting my time?"

each other. This building of trust decreases judgment and fear of another's assumed ill-intent.

In these pages, we are going to talk about fear and about strategies for combatting compassion fatigue and burnout, which can cause good staff to lose hope and motivation, to walk out of a job, or leave the healthcare field entirely.

The suggestions for the days and weeks to follow are offered as a catalyst to open the doors of opportunity for more positive communication, sharing, being fully present, and experiencing the range of events that compassion brings.

We have to do things in ways we've never done them, and we need to take some risks with the anticipation of high rewards in terms of human connection. We need to be sensitive to those for whom this is bold thinking and unfamiliar territory, because they see compassion and business as distinct subjects that should not appear in the same sentence, as separate as oil and water. This is how we will learn from and about each other and overcome differences as well as make a difference.

Are hospitals, clinics, nursing homes, medical offices, assisted living communities, and other health-care providers willing to announce that the next step beyond caring—compassion—is a fully functioning and active component in their care environments for all departments and all levels of staff? If not, why? What are they afraid of?

A culture and practice of compassionate ways provides a bridge, a history upon which to communicate, share, and connect in challenging times. That is the solution and the goal.

28 Ways of Compassionate People: LEAD

The 28 ways are simple and relatively straightforward. For ease of understanding for the reader they are grouped into four directives: Listen, Engage, Act, and Dare to Care (LEAD). These directives are easily applied to a seven-day week or to a twenty-eight-day cycle. This is a commonly accepted timeframe to start creating the foundation of new habits and behaviors.

We all know, unfortunately, that *simple* doesn't always equate to *easy*. Along with being afraid, people have been unwilling and unable to constructively discuss the topic of compassion in the workplace. There has been a lack of direction, a lack of protocol, and a lack of knowledge about HOW to discuss it.

What we need is doing—*action*—achieved through practice, practice, and more practice. Deep and lasting transformation happens in tiny increments: actions practiced over time, day by day, minute by minute.

By choosing to take action, each of us can give a more positive human experience of health care to our patients and coworkers through the organizations we serve. To be sure, the actions, tools, and techniques shared in this book can be used in many other scenarios beyond healthcare. Opportunities to improve and enhance communications and relations occur naturally throughout our personal and work lives—including "work" in any industry or setting. Human connections are central to our life experience, period. This book is about strengthening and maximizing the connection opportunities that we have every single day. Because at the end of the day, that's what life is about: Those connections are where the magic happens.

28 Ways of Compassion is not asking you to do anything that you are not already capable of doing. It asks you to look differently at your interactions and the way you work and live and make tiny changes with a rich potential payoff.

You have nothing to lose, and yet you have everything to gain.

Listen

We become receptive to the wealth of
information that is offered to us in our day.

We are open to communication from
unusual or unexpected sources.

We benefit from being more accurately
informed and aware.

1.

Use More Than
the Ears to Listen

"To listen fully means to pay close attention to what is being
said beneath the words. You listen not only to the 'music,' but to
the essence of the person speaking. You listen not only for what
someone knows, but for what he or she is. Ears operate at the speed
of sound, which is far slower than the speed of light the eyes take
in. Generative listening is the art of developing deeper silences in
yourself, so you can slow your mind's hearing to your ears' natural
speed, and hear beneath the words to their meaning."

—PETER SENGE

Communication is the number one responsibility of being a
leader. It is the top priority.

To the people you lead, you are the most important person in
the company. The success of these people and their commitment

to the workplace are completely dependent on the quality and effectiveness of their direct relationship, their connection, with you. Employees stay with or leave their supervisor, not the company.

A survey of twenty thousand employees done by Comparably, a compensation, culture, and jobs monitoring site, found that manager communication was the skill most in need of improvement. Fully half of the respondents listed it as the top issue.[1]

The key component of any successful communication is listening. The challenge is learning how to practice listening more effectively in order to be better at communicating.

We can begin by learning to "hear" with more than just our ears, to listen deeply, fully, and totally and take in all of the information available to us. When you're a leader, people watch and listen to you with close attention, even when you think they're not, because it affects them. You do the same with your leaders. Whether it's a direct or indirect leadership relationship, people gather information from your facial expression, your tone, and the volume of your voice; those sources of information are at least equal to any words you might say

I was the HR director for a large inbound call center, where more than five hundred operators provided service to Spiegel catalog customers. Rumors of lay-offs started circulating, rumors that were not true. When I traced the

---

1   "STUDY: How People Really Feel About Their Bosses," Comparably.com, July 14, 2017, https://www.comparably.com/blog/study-bosses/.

source, I found out that one of the reps had seen me with a distressed, unhappy face walking across the call center floor. For her, it was a sure sign that bad news was on the way. Thinking back, I told her it had been a severe stomach ache. The point is, she was "listening" to my face and making up information to match it.

We are all born to listen. While we're in our mother's womb, we tune in to the sounds of her body and the noises of her world: voices, music, cars, animals, phones, television. Although newborns are not able to comprehend language, they instinctively understand and are calmed by soft tones and soothing vibrations, and they react with a startle reflex to sharp, abrupt, and loud sounds.

The newborn is like a little sponge. Babies connect with us through all five senses to try to understand the new world around them. Most babies are born with the ability to hear, along with the ability to feel (touch), taste, and smell. But newborns can only focus their eyesight 8–15 inches away for the first month, and then the distance increases to about three feet; only later does human eyesight reach its full range. Making eye contact is extremely important for the baby, so much so, in fact, that they want to look at both eyes, not just one. They intently study the faces, sounds, and motions of their caretakers, gaining meaning and emotion without language.

It's not until about two months that babies start to respond and interact, replying to messages they receive from us with a smile, a gurgle, or an outstretched hand. Babies want to make use of as much information as possible, so they *listen* with everything they have.

Fast forward to adulthood and the world of work. We have, over time, decreased some of our earlier sensitivity to the non-verbal clues around us. We may limit our attention more to what people actually say, the words, than we do to the expressions, the body language, the information-rich clues available through our other senses. We're able to talk between closed doors, on the phone, and look down or multitask during face-to-face conversations, and thus we fail to give our full attention to the communication source. By becoming so skilled with spoken and written language, we're not listening with all of our senses. We don't feel the need to spend energy to hear as thoroughly as we used to.

We need to recognize that any given conversation or interaction with someone in our world of work may be of extreme importance to them, whether they are a coworker, staff member, customer, or patient. They are listening to us very attentively, even when we think they aren't. And they want to be heard, totally. It is a basic human need to be heard and, hopefully, in turn understood. No amount of work that we do to train or formalize communication processes will fix it if people feel that we aren't fully listening.

What can you expect when your listening improves? For starters, by practicing compassionate listening your valuable time will be more effectively utilized because you'll be fully present, engaged, and receptive. People's level of comfort and confidence in you will grow as you build credibility as a caring individual who listens fully.

You'll build trust within your staff, teams, and the patients or residents that you serve. You may even find that this trust and confidence lowers anxiety and tension and repeated requests for attention.

Finally, where there's no listening, there's no understanding. No understanding means no compassion, and no compassion means there's no connection. It all starts with real listening. That's why this is the first way—or exercise—and first section. To begin to plant the seeds of compassion at work you have to listen with more than your ears. You have to listen with your heart.

Exercises for Day 1

· Pay mindful attention to total listening. Listen with your face, your eyes, and your body language. As a start, if at all possible, when meeting with people, close your office door, don't answer your phone, and provide a private space. Consider sitting with your back to your office windows to minimize your chance of distraction.

· For scheduled conversations, make a brief bullet list of items that must be covered so you can fully engage with your senses during the meeting. Refer to your list as needed and before drawing the session to a close.

· If interrupted while working on a paper project, mark your spot with your finger or a pencil. If you feel you should set the project aside temporarily, wrap up your thought, mark your

continued

35

place, and focus your attention on this new matter at hand. The person will feel heard and acknowledged.

· If you're interrupted during a hallway, office, or breakroom conversation (as we often are), take a quick moment to say to the first person, "Please excuse me a moment," before responding to the person who has approached you. This shows respect and compassion for the needs of both individuals, and they both will notice it. Then direct your attention where it is most needed.

--------- **Reflections** ---------

Now consider these questions:

1. How would my staff rate me as a listener? Do they feel *heard* by me?

2. What, if anything, distracted me from listening as well as I could today?

3. Describe a situation today where listening better helped me.

4. What are three things I can do tomorrow to listen better than I did today?

2.

Share Joy with the Sadness

"Joy is always an integral part of loving. There is joy in every act
of life, no matter how menial or repetitive. To work in love is
to work in joy. To live in love is to live in joy . . .
Why not choose joy? . . . Why not live in joy?"

—LEO BUSCAGLIA

It's a typical Monday morning, and staff are gathering in a small
conference room for a weekly meeting. Some of those who've
arrived a little early are taking the opportunity to review their
to-do lists and calendars. Others are chatting among themselves,
sharing stories of events that happened over the weekend.

As the meeting leader joins the group, one nurse, Susie, is
sharing how happy she is that her daughter's long-planned wed-
ding went off without a hitch. With a slight smile, the leader
glances around the room, sits down, and asks, "Everyone here?
Good, let's get started."

Suddenly the happy mood vanishes, and Susie doesn't get to finish her great news. Conversation ceases, attention turns to the work at hand.

Is there anything horribly wrong with this scenario? Not really. But does something feel not quite right? Yes, maybe. There was a real opportunity for the leader to show that she was paying attention, that she cares, and she wants to connect. Susie was talking to her team, which includes the leader, about a big, happy, and important event in her life. She was inviting the group to share it with her. A positive moment went unrecognized and ignored, probably leaving Susie feeling unheard.

But isn't this book about compassion, and doesn't compassion mean sharing and empathizing with bad, sad things?

For the purposes of this book, and the interpretation of the word compassion that we're using, we're going to believe that compassion is broader than sadness and suffering.

It *is* about feelings and emotions. It *is* about what's going on now, in the moment. But we are not going to limit our definition to things that are bad or sad, or limit our compassionate ways to situations where mercy or pity is bestowed by one person onto another. We're going to expand the scope of our compassion to encompass all feelings and all happenings—happy, sad, sweet, funny, surprising, shocking, or whatever that feeling may be.

Honestly, when we look at definitions of the word, they typically talk about sympathy, empathy, victims, mercy, or pity; being concerned for the misfortunes of others; desiring to help someone who's sick, hungry, or in trouble; or wanting to alleviate the pain of another. Because the word *passion* derives from a Greek word meaning "suffering" and the prefix *com* means "together," it is most often described as involving some type of "suffering together."

In my study of compassionate people and their ways, however, I saw behavior that went beyond sad to happy, even in the very worst of times. I saw compassion where people were immersed in the present, open in their expression, and striving with every conceivable part of themselves to make a genuine connection with another human.

Let's agree to agree that *com* means "together." Then let's consider this definition of *passion* that I found by chance in *The Urban Dictionary*: "Passion is when you put more energy into something than is required to do it. It is more than just enthusiasm or excitement, passion is ambition that is materialized into action to put as much heart, mind, body, and soul into something as is possible."

This view of "together passion" doesn't say anything about good or bad or happy or sad. It says that we will be prompted by something to take strong, motivated action. We'll put more than just minimal effort into this something. We'll give it our full attention. Yes, in the work world, including the field of healthcare, we often are dealing with negative, uncomfortable, and even tragic circumstances that require our full effort and deep levels of compassion. We can sometimes become blinded to the positive, so that it becomes almost a nonexistent "something." Some might even think that in our stressful, critical environments it's disrespectful to celebrate together the good things that are happening around us.

When we make a choice to participate in happy moments

with people, even in sad circumstances such as when a loved one is recovering in a hospital, it is not disrespectful. In fact, sharing that something funny, amusing, or special has happened is a way of saying that we are engaged, listening, and connecting with the person. It shows that we see the person as a person and that we can handle all the shades of life in healthcare and leadership.

It was the fall of 1998, and my husband was trying to cheer up our daughter while she was hospitalized for chemotherapy treatment. She was the first child to be admitted to the oncology unit at Renown in Reno, so she was surrounded on the floor by adult patients. She was receiving an infusion over several days but had a portable IV pole and was able to walk around with the infusion bags hanging from its side.

Because it was around Halloween time, my husband got the crazy idea to take an empty hydration bag, put some dry ice in it, and add a little water. So as Denae was taking her walk on the oncology floor that night, patients in other rooms, visitors, and the nurses watched with wide eyes as a trail of bubbly cloudy mist drifted along the pole to the floor and disappeared down the hallway.

Many laughed, some simply stared, and one patient asked, "What chemo drugs is she on?" The nurses thought it was pretty funny! But there was one grumpy nurse who criticized the fun: "I thought the child was going to be a problem, but it's her parents." Hmpf!

We all want a nurse who smiles and laughs with us instead of turning us away. We want a boss who writes a personal note in the circulated birthday card or thanks us for our service with a special story or shares a good word or congratulations about something they heard we are celebrating. Shared happiness is more fun! We want people with us when we're happy, someone to share our joys with, just as we do our hardships. That's the full realization of compassion.

Exercises for Day 2

Try to do at least two of these three exercises before the end of the day:

- Look online and in various dictionaries at definitions and descriptions related to the word *compassion*. Make notes in the section at the end of this chapter about the words that are related to feelings. This should help you better understand the purpose behind this chapter: to get you thinking in broader terms about the word and the action of compassion itself.

- Talk with others you encounter today about what compassion means to them. Ask patients, residents, coworkers, your boss, maybe even a stranger with whom you strike up a conversation.

- Keep your radar alert and your ear to the ground for happy moments occurring or being talked about around you today. Don't be like the team leader in the story at the beginning of this segment. Grab any chance to model compassionate action.

——————————— **Reflections** ———————————

1. What words did I find in the dictionary to describe the word *compassion*?

2. What words or definitions did other people share with me?

3. Here's a happy moment I came across, and here are thoughts I have about it.

4. How do I feel differently about compassion now than I did before this chapter?

3.

Look Past Blame

"Great leaders don't rush to blame.
They instinctively look for solutions."

—NINA EASTON

Of the many ways that miscommunication can hurt a situation, the quick pinpointing and placing of blame when something has gone wrong is arguably one of the worst.

You hurry through your workday, complete your to-do lists and tasks, and then BAM! you're confronted with staff issues, errors, and miscommunications. In short, you have to deal with problems that seem like inconveniences to your productivity. It might be tempting to take in only as much new information as you think you need to know, use what you think you already know about the situation or the person, and then consider what's been done in the past. Based on this you can come to a decision about what happened, who did it, and what to do to fix it quickly. Right?

Wrong. Every situation is unique to itself, every person, and every interaction. It's crucial that you begin with a blank screen and allow each detail to come in new and fresh. Look at it from several angles, keep asking the question why rather than who. Beyond focusing just on what happened, move to finding out how and why it happened. Do this with each situation. Only when we've answered these questions can we go back to the start and consider new options for this and future occurrences.

Our minds want to put closure to problems, obstacles, questions, and riddles. But the most obvious or logical solution is not necessarily the correct one. In healthcare and leadership we cannot afford to be wrong in identifying causes and effects. At stake are people's lives and livelihoods, or at the very least people's reputations. In a case where we wrongly blame and punish an employee, it devastates the employee and has huge morale and monetary costs to the organization. In a case where we blame a patient for issues with their care, claiming they're difficult or they're noncompliant, we may be missing the real cause of a complication.

You must invest adequate time in each issue's beginning, clear your mind, and approach challenging investigations with fresh eyes and few preconceived notions. These thoughtful actions will pay dividends later when you're not wasting time rehashing the same problem, draining your energies in the wrong direction, and backtracking as you find out new facts that you should have asked about in the first place.

When people learn that this is how you operate, that you're not on a mission to place blame, they will be more open about what's really happening. They won't be so afraid of being blamed.

You need to always be painstakingly thorough and careful in assigning blame. You need to eliminate the words *blame* and *fault* from your work conversations and replace them with words like *cause, solution, correction, truth,* and *fact.*

Again, when in doubt, keep asking why. Then how, what, when, and where. Who is the least important. In fact, knowing names may actually cloud people's judgment and get them jumping to conclusions based on wrong facts.

Compassion has no place for blame.

Exercises for Day 3

- Consider: Are you someone who looks to place blame? If so, do you place blame quickly or slowly? Look at recent events, then pay mindful attention today to the behavior of yourself and others on your team.

- Observe whether others feel comfortable discussing problem situations with you. Check whether you're open to what they're saying.

- Watch for ample space for people to question and respond thoroughly. You should be modeling the way. Don't give them the solution; help them come to a reasonable plan.

- If people come to you with guilty verdicts, blaming someone, stop them in their tracks and redirect them.

Reflections
---

1. Briefly describe the first case that comes to your mind where you or someone else jumped to blame and was wrong.

2. How does *not* jumping to blame or faulting someone make you a better leader, coworker, or caregiver? List at least three ways.

3. Could your team or company adopt a "no blame, only solutions" philosophy?

4.

Choose When to Cross Boundaries

"The sky has never been the limit. We have our own limits.
It is then about breaking our personal limit and
outgrowing ourselves to live our best life."

—DR. ANIL KUMAR SINHA

In the world of work we're often told, "Keep it strictly business," "Don't get personally involved," and "Leave your emotions at the door."

In contrast, we're also instructed to be caring. We tell our staff to be caring. Yet we aren't told and don't effectively guide or model to our staff how to be caring, what it looks and feels like, and where the boundaries lie. As a result, we sometimes function well within the safe zone and hesitate to get closer to others at work, or we jump way out beyond the safety net and set ourselves up for not only inappropriate interactions but also burnout and compassion fatigue.

So this concept of moving from a passive role of *having* caring and compassion to an active role of *showing* compassion and *practicing* compassionate ways at work can be an uncomfortable proposition.

Why? Because it is unfamiliar territory, full of unknowns, and could mean a loss of control. It can make the idea of exercising compassion something that an aspiring or current leader doesn't want to consider, even though the leader may know that he needs better communication and connection with his workforce if he's going to be effective and if he's going to have a chance of being extraordinary.

Because this constitutes a barrier to growth, it is a pain point, something that we need to talk about and get past if we're to keep moving forward. Let's be honest and brave!

The answer isn't easy, but it is simple. It's this: Authentic, caring, and compassionate people are comfortable with being uncomfortable. They're not on guard against the unknown, and they let themselves be vulnerable. They can be this way because they have developed a level of confidence that comes from being clear about what their personal and professional boundaries are and honoring them.

It's this awareness and thoughtful practice that lets real, compassionate people feel uncomfortable while holding on to a measure of control. They know how far their discomfort can reasonably extend.

For myself, I've realized that sometimes I hold back, shutting off my feelings and compassion because I'm afraid that I'll get pulled in too deep. I worry that I might sacrifice some degree of restraint, discretion, or judgment and won't be able to regain it.

When I open up without being prepared and others unexpectedly cross my boundaries it feels, well, awful. The sense of safety floating away creates a tangible experience of loss. The best way I can describe the emotion is regret and personal failure. I feel I've let myself get "sucked in" and promised—or worse—given away more than I intended. When I feel that someone has taken advantage of me, my reaction is to want to close off. Hurting, I tell myself that maybe I shouldn't risk being open again. The other person may be left confused and hurt as well, not knowing what they did wrong and why I've withdrawn.

The remedy to this flip-flop between totally open or completely closed off is to start building a mindful awareness of what early discomfort feels like. You can do this by listening carefully to your body, mind, and heart. You need to learn what comfort feels like before you can recognize discomfort. Then you'll need to continue practicing self-awareness, slowing down, taking a breath, and naming feelings and emotions as they come up. Understand that you do have choices. This is how you can begin to uncover and shore up your own personal boundaries.

This important exercise will shape your connections as you progress through the book. We all have boundaries. You need to learn to trust yourself and know that you won't "lose control" so you can feel safe getting closer to another person. Don't overpromise, try to solve someone else's problem beyond what you're capable of, take on more than you are thoughtfully willing to take, give another even more than they ask for, be inconsistent or unfair between people, or compromise your own work or home situation for their benefit.

You can still get caught off guard and find yourself facing yet another unknown in the midst of a hectic, demanding workday. When I have those days I try to step into an empty cubby or the restroom or basically any space that I can pretend is a sanctuary for a moment. I tell myself a quick affirmation that goes something like this: "Honor yourself, Dee, and honor those around you." I take a long, deep breath and end with a smile that I imagine pushing into my heart. This might sound strange to you, but don't dismiss it until you've tried it.

Being mindful about your boundaries and intentions will help get you to a place that is real and authentic, a safe, compassionate place for you and others. Your boundaries are well worth maintaining and nurturing to keep you healthy.

Exercises for Day 4

- Go into today's home and work situations with your compassionate self. Acknowledge any discomfort and take baby steps.

- Pay attention to how you're feeling. Take note of those happenings where you feel like you're entering unfamiliar or uncomfortable territory.

- Notice if there are times that you held back when you might have had an urge to do or share more with someone. It could be something as simple as a passing smile in a hallway or a comment that you let go by that may have been an opening or attempt to talk. Why did you hold back?

- If you can, determine your intentions for any upcoming personal meetings. Outline what you hope to achieve and how far you'll go to get there. Write down what you are not willing to compromise or give up, ever.

Reflections

---

1. What situations, if any, caused you discomfort today?

2. What would you need to overcome before you could be more open and compassionate at work?

5.

Adapt to the Different Ways That People Learn

"For the things we have to learn before we can do them,
we learn by doing them."

—ARISTOTLE

You can't study compassion without studying how people learn. No matter what your specific discipline is, you perform training in your work roles. Do you think of yourself as a trainer? Have you been taught how to train? If your job title doesn't include the words *trainer*, *educator*, or *instructor*, then probably not.

Unless education is your profession, I doubt that you've ever learned much about how to train or how people learn. To be successful in passing along critical knowledge to the staff and patients or residents in your community, however, you must understand some basics about training and the learning process.

The first step is to recognize, first and foremost, that all people learn differently. Your training success and your ability to achieve the goals set out for you are highly dependent on how much you pay attention to what makes people tick. You need to discover how your individual people learn best and adapt your training to them.

If you don't feel like a trainer, consider this: Every time you communicate with another person you are teaching them something that is new. Yes, this is a big claim. But even if you say, "Hi, how are you?" you're modeling your expected standard of behavior and your culture.

Regardless of our professional title, we're all training constantly, whenever we share information one-on-one, in groups, verbally, in writing, in hands-on demonstrations, or letting someone know something they did not know before. It could be a procedure, policy, or protocol. It could be an update, or it might be feedback. It might be orienting new staff, being a buddy to a coworker, supervising care, reporting to a shift manager, or giving discharge instructions to a patient. All of these qualify as training.

When you are responsible for training of any type you should be asking yourself this question: How well was the knowledge received? Just because you provide training, how do you know that the information was understood in the manner it was intended and that the purpose of this knowledge was clear? In truth, if the "student" isn't learning, then you're not teaching. How often have you heard someone say, "They received training in that" after another person makes an error? If a person doesn't know how to do their job correctly then they didn't learn, regardless of what training was administered.

Training may be designed as a one-size-fits-all application, but it's not received that way and learning doesn't happen that way. Learning is person-centric, meaning it's individual to the person's style and abilities. A good example of this type of learning is in the field of special education. The overall academic goals may be similar to those of mainstream classrooms. However, each child has an individualized education plan, with the teacher aware of the plans and adapting strategies to each student. Care is taken to check frequently for comprehension and to use alternate methods of delivering the training if a particular one is seen to be ineffective.

In special education, if a student is not achieving the desired results, the instructor adjusts to the student, not the other way around. We need to work with our staff and others in the same way, delivering the knowledge in a way that works best for them.

All staff should be given basic instruction on how to effectively train others. If that's not possible, at a bare minimum all healthcare staff need to understand that each person learns best through hearing, seeing, doing, or any combination of these. Overall retention improves when a variety of methods are used.

Practicing compassion will naturally complement person-centered training. If the teacher is focused on the learner and his needs, and is truly trying to understand and relate to the other person (as compassionate people do), then teaching becomes a completely individual, one-of-a-kind event. It is another way you can genuinely engage with the uniqueness you find across the diversity of your workforce.

The payoff for these efforts is that you can spend less time repeating training, and you can be more confident in the quality of care when staff and patients truly understand what they need to know.

Exercises for Day 5

- Tell yourself several times today, "I am a teacher." Make yourself believe it.

- Consider this statement today: Communication is a process, not an event. The same applies to training. Recognize the education portion of every action you take.

- Next time you do formal training, focus attention on the reactions of the other person or the audience. Invite questions and reflection. Ask: "Can I try to explain or show this another way so you can understand it better?" Every second and every question you allow is going to save you time and misunderstanding in the end.

———————————— **Reflections** ————————————

1. How did being aware that information is received differently affect any of your interactions today?

2. Which way(s) do you think that you learn best?

3. How do you know?

6.

Have Flexibility in Response to Interruptions

"Don't let goal setting become heavy weights.
Remain flexible and allow room for intuitive changes."

—KELLY MARTIN

How many interruptions—oops—I mean conversations in your day start with the question, "Do you have a minute?"

When I was the HR Director for a large health system, frequent interruptions and the "minutes that turn into a half hour" had become a source of voiced frustration among members of my senior leadership team. They were coming to me as a mediator of sorts, complaining about the lack of respect and consideration being shown for their time. They needed a polite way to send a direct message without hurting anyone's feelings or causing conflicts. We agreed to a plan, and I introduced a tool under a session titled "Real

Time Management" in our monthly Boot Camp leadership development meeting. I gave each director a one-minute sand timer and guidance on how to use it. When someone approached them in their office and asked, "Do you have a minute?" the answer was, as they turned over the sand timer and smiled, "Why yes I do!" The action was friendly and to the point. Everyone liked the idea because it cleared the air while sending the message it was intended to send. In circumstances when more time was needed, the expectation was talked about up front. It worked very well.

There are a couple of considerations to be aware of as you respond to people who ask for your time: respect for each person and the frequency of the event.

Sometimes the asker is presuming that the answer will be yes. Everyone has a minute, so many of us find it difficult to say no. Sometimes what the asker wants to discuss is important and urgent; sometimes it isn't. It sometimes has something to do with them putting their needs before yours, and you letting them. If this is the case, it is an interruption, which is inconvenient. The deeper problem here is that when we're chronically interrupted for not-so-critical matters it makes it more difficult for the crucial ones to get our attention.

It's like the story of the boy who cried wolf so often that people began to ignore him—then one day there really was a wolf. Those who truly need us can be drowned out by those who continually demand our attention. This was illustrated to me very strongly one day when I found myself reflexively saying,

"Not right now" to someone who asked if I had a minute. It was the most horrible feeling in the world when they explained that there had been a sudden death in the family, and they needed my immediate help with time off work. I would rather say yes a hundred times and be inconvenienced than say no ever again and be wrong.

Wayne Dyer said, and I believe, "Miracles come in moments. Be ready and willing." You must always be attentive to and really listen to every person who approaches you for your time. By taking just a moment—usually it's less—to focus totally on who is asking, their demeanor, and their approach, you should be able to judge how critical the issue might be.

A thoughtful response shows that you've heard them, and that you're not going to simply dismiss any request from someone who wants to see you. People learn to respect that you may really not have the time right then. If you're working on something for someone else, the asker will know that when their concern comes up, you'll be treating it with the same dedicated attention. These actions build trust. People want to know you care, and it doesn't matter how much you say you do if you don't show it when it truly matters. Leading is caring.

You'll benefit from having open discussions about time and availability with your teammates and staff. You should respect, understand, and have compassion for the responsibilities others carry. Remember to consider the demands you make of others' time just as you would like them to be sensitive to yours.

Exercises for Day 6

- The next time someone asks you if you have a moment or asks if they can talk to you, look at them, consider how they approached you, and consider who they are. Even if you're busy, ask if it's something that can wait before you answer. Depending on the response, you can then say one of two things: "Yes, I have _____ minutes. What can I do for you?" or "I'm so sorry, but I don't right now. Can we get together _____?"

- Remember that listening for understanding is the key.

Reflections

1. How much did interruptions interfere with my day today?

2. What plan could I make to handle them better, so I can be responsive when someone really needs me?

3. Do my work teams have an issue with overusing the question "Do you have a minute?" If so, could the teams work together on different ways to address it?

7.

Believe in Making a Difference

"What you do makes a difference, and you have to decide what kind of difference you want to make."

—JANE GOODALL

You may feel like you've accomplished little at the end of a task-filled day. Your to-do list may seem as long as it was at the beginning of the day. You may be tired and frazzled and feel like your wheels have been spinning wildly for hours, but you didn't move anywhere.

Without a doubt, healthcare is one of the most rewarding yet challenging fields in which to work. Whether we are in a front-line role interacting directly with the customer, or we serve behind the scenes, supporting the front line by managing and organizing to keep everything running as it should, we all have an impact on people's lives. Every day.

It can be really hard to see that unless we choose to look for it. Here is a text my daughter, a sonographer, shared with me recently:

"I have worked really, really, REALLY hard and sacrificed a lot to finish school and follow this path that I've always wanted, and I LOVE what I do. It's not always pretty and a lot of days are hard and I see sad stuff happen to good people. I'd say a good 95 percent of the scans I do in a day are pointless, and the person has nothing wrong with them. But to have someone tell me I made a difference just with my bright smile. Or to draw a picture for a little kid I just sent to surgery that makes him stop crying. It's all worth it. I've found things on six patients this week that probably saved their lives. And it feels good to every once in a while feel like I'm making a difference, that I am doing good. Thank you for always believing in me."

Here's the truth. We are all, always, making a difference. Sometimes the difference we make is in being—being totally present where we are and being the best we can at any given moment. We might not see it because we're so focused on the doing. Know this: Even the smallest positive effort accomplishes more than no effort. We are all making things happen.

This book is directed not only at direct clinical care providers and executives in the healthcare industry, but also at all the staff who work in this field. That's right, we are all "make-things-happen people": dishwashers, groundskeepers, CNAs (Certified Nursing Assistants), accountants, CEOs, housekeepers. We keep things moving and happening when we are where we are supposed to be, when we are supposed to be there. We may be way out of sight, but we are nevertheless vital to the community in which we serve. Think of a duck on a pond, looking so still and serene as it moves across the water. Not much seems to be happening, right? But under the water the duck's little feet are working away, doing their job, one little paddle not making a huge difference, but both together, look at that duck go! Each positive action of our team is doing the same, moving the organization forward, making things a little better, fulfilling the mission and propelling us toward our future.

It's important that we see it and believe it. You were put in each moment for a reason.

Exercises for Day 7

- Today know that you are making a difference. Take note of how you're changing your environment. Are you making the kind of difference you want to make? Note whether it is a positive one.

- Be aware of opportunities and do what only you can do in the moment. You'll get other chances, but you won't get the exact same chance again. Concentrate on NOW.

continued

- Pay attention! Open a door, smile, write a thank you note, take a moment to listen.

- Draw a picture for that little boy going to surgery.

--- **Reflections** ---

1. Why am I in this job? What am I supposed to "make happen" in the lives of other people?

2. What are three things I made happen today?

3. How do I feel about my ability to make a difference after this lesson and today's prompts? Do I believe that I make a difference? Why or why not?

Engage

We choose to move beyond listening
and observing to become a participant
who is actively invested in the
happenings around us.

We create an increased sense of energy
within ourselves and those with whom
we interact.

The environment becomes more alive
and purpose-driven.

8.

Bring the Full Self
to Every Encounter

"When you love someone, the best thing you can offer is your
presence. How can you love if you are not there?"

—THICH NHAT HANH

We feel so busy at work, how can we possibly muster the time and
energy to be *more* engaged, *more* involved, and *more* participative
with our staff? We can't make any more hours in the day. We're
booked solid with meetings, paperwork, consultations, project
work, phone calls, plus interruptions, and the list goes on. We
can't be any more places than we already are.

But the fact is, we aren't always where we are! Think about
it. Aren't there times when you're physically present in a given
location—heart beating, eyes open, breathing in and out. You
could even be doing activities that require real focus or be engaged

in a face-to-face conversation, but, by some feat of nature, you may not be present mentally. Your body is there, moving on some version of autopilot, but your mind is traveling around, visiting what happened an hour ago, yesterday, last year. Or you may be contemplating the future, making plans, thinking about events that may or may not happen.

This kind of absence became crystal clear to me a couple of years ago. Maybe you've heard the common postcard greeting, "Beautiful! Wish you were here!" I was at a breathtakingly gorgeous viewpoint on the top of a mountain in Antigua, West Indies, but in my head I was reviewing a to-do list for the next week. It struck me that I wasn't there mentally. I laughed and said out loud, with my arms outstretched, "Beautiful! Wish I was here!" It's become a great reminder, to me, to be where I am.

Transfer this concept of being fully present or engaged into the work setting. For a long time, the business world focused on measuring the satisfaction levels of staff and correlated those levels with company success. However, in recent decades, businesses have come to understand that staff engagement, or the level of presence and commitment, has a more significant impact on the performance potential of the teams and the organization as a whole. This engagement is also highly associated with the proactivity and involvement of the leaders. So how engaged are you with your staff? How much are you truly interacting, applying your discretionary effort, showing people by example the behavior you expect from them?

Our daily work provides chances to connect with others in a

variety of ways. Our success as leaders relies on recognizing and understanding the potential in each of these moments. If we aren't fully present then we are missing the opportunity right in front of us to make the difference that I believe each of us wants to make.

It is the greatest of human desires to be fully seen, heard, and understood. The word *intimacy* is sometimes broken down to a simple definition of "into me, see." When surveyed by organizations a frequent top issue with employees is that their leadership does not listen to, understand, or respond to their needs.

It is a willingness to be present, to really see, to engage that separates extraordinary leaders from the rest. People who feel understood, seen, and heard feel part of something bigger, feel a sense of belonging. They develop enough trust and confidence in leaders to follow them because they believe that leadership cares about their needs and concerns. If there is no trust then there is no connection and no progress. And an opportunity to move forward together has been missed.

Don't waste the moments. It will take no additional time or energy to be present, to participate, and to engage.

Exercises for Day 8

- Commit right now that you will check in with yourself frequently to ask, "Am I here?"

- Whenever you find yourself absent, get centered. Bring yourself into the here and now. Do this by simply taking a deep breath

continued

and becoming totally aware of your surroundings. Ask yourself three questions:

What am I doing?

Who am I with?

Why am I here?

· With practice this will become a natural habit.

· Wherever you are, go there! Show up! Be there!

Reflections

1. How many times today did I catch myself being absent?

2. What happened?

3. How glad am I that I did this exercise? What did I learn?

4. What can I do tomorrow to stay better focused?

9.

Practice Being Open

"The way to make people trust-worthy is to trust them."
—ERNEST HEMINGWAY

In business we have a lot of experience closing ourselves off, even being guarded. But making real connections requires that we be open. Our ability to communicate in meaningful ways is dependent on the quality of these connections. We have to be open to recognize and act on opportunities for connection. Openness must be practiced, and openness requires that we risk letting down some of our shields.

Human beings are wired to be open. We build our walls and screens as a protection out of fear. People would rather feel nothing than feel pain, uncertainty, and sadness. Closing ourselves off is safe and predictable, but in doing so we miss so much.

It's simple to grasp that your senses would be lessened with cotton balls stuffed in your ears, a blindfold over your eyes, a clip on your nose, or gloves on your hands. These are examples of physical blocks. With these physical blocks, you might still experience faint sensation, but the experience in the moment would be dulled at best. With these blocks, you wouldn't be fully aware of what was happening around you.

Similarly, you might choose to keep yourself removed from others in a physical way. Maybe you stay in your office rather than interact, or you remain "separate" by not listening fully, disregarding stimuli you're receiving, using distractions, or holding back personal thoughts or insights that might be helpful. In other words, disengaging.

If you're going to attract and complete the connections that will transform any moment of communication into an opportunity for real sharing, then you have to be open. Think of it as taking off the gloves.

Taking off the gloves—opening up—will make you more vulnerable, but it doesn't mean you're ignoring your boundaries. You will still choose when to enhance connections by sharing who you are and becoming real and three dimensional.

As with swimming, riding a bicycle, and driving a car, talking about opening up and reading about it are not doing it. It takes awareness, practice, patience with oneself, and above all, time to learn to open yourself to others. You will have to be vigilant to notice when you're putting a protective guard between yourself and a person or situation. When we can selectively choose openness and proceed unguarded, we can feel the beginnings of connections that may grow into better caring, understanding, and compassion.

This book is designed so that you *can* practice the actions in daily doses and experience some of the thoughts and feelings that happen when you are openly compassionate. Being openly compassionate allows others a glimpse inside of you and invites them to approach you and build trust, to make a connection.

Approachability is a key trait of extraordinary leaders. People often ask, "How do I make myself more approachable?" This chapter contains the roadmap for practicing the openness that will get you there.

Being approachable will open you up to many more opportunities to connect with people during your day. Others may not react immediately. In my experience, it can take a couple of times, or the other person may take a couple of days to get up the nerve to approach you. But I'm confident that you will open doors to communication that may have been closed or maybe just ajar.

Being a leader means being, not just doing. Leading is about influence, not control. Leaders inspire trust and confidence. They model the behavior they want to see. They are champions of the change they wish to drive. Through doing today's activities you will realize that you're naturally creating the connections you need to be a successful leader.

Exercises for Day 9

- Start with taking a deep, slow breath. Think about where you are right now, in this second. Listen to the sounds around you and observe every little thing that's happening. Look with fresh eyes, as if it's the first time you're in your surroundings. Do this several times during the day to bring yourself into the current moment.

- Each time you take a deep, slow breath, think about being open physically. What's your body doing? Uncross your arms. Lighten up your expression/soften your face and your gaze. Relax your facial muscles. Open up your chest. Feel openness.

- Here's a big order for the day: Spend more time alone. This may seem the opposite of everything I just said, but I don't mean spend time alone in your office. What I mean is to be alone yet available to others. Alone/available in the hallway, elevator, restroom, after a meeting. Linger! Have a cup of coffee alone. Allow yourself to travel around without someone with you, and be approachable with your face, eyes, and body. Walk with your head up and make eye contact and greet people that you pass.

Reflections

1. Describe ways that you allowed yourself to take off your gloves today.

2. How did you participate more fully in meetings or other interactions?

3. If you did the "alone and available" stretch exercise, did you have any interesting encounters? *Note:* Give it time. Practice. People need to get acquainted with a different you and gain confidence in their ability to trust you.

10.

Believe in the Best
of Each Person

"Individuals make impressions and judgments about people
very quickly, very easily, and with minimal information.
And once those judgments are made, they tend to be
hard to undo. They're quite sticky."

—DR. VIVIAN ZAYAS, ASSOCIATE PROFESSOR,
CORNELL UNIVERSITY

It's human nature to subconsciously take in the information
that is available to us and make decisions about people based on
this data. It's estimated that we form a first impression based on
outward appearances alone in as little as five seconds. Then our
impression is molded by *how* a person talks, and *then* what they
say. How we perceive and understand them is determined by
these narrow judgments. Unless we choose to be more aware of

and explore these possible unconscious biases, and become more open to and inclusive of further information, our actions could be founded in false beliefs.

The false belief may lean toward the positive, such as believing someone is competent because they look competent, or the negative, such as assuming that a disheveled, unorganized person is a slacker.

When it leans to the negative, it can limit the possibilities of what we see in them. People often will live up to our expectations of them. Assuming the worst of people rather than seeing and encouraging their best results in missed opportunities and lessens our chances for success and happiness.

Recently I had the experience of avoiding even the possibility of meeting a certain public person. I'm ashamed to say it, even to myself, but it was totally about my discomfort. I had made assumptions about his personality and character that were based on my own personal beliefs and experiences with people who looked and presented like him. So I removed myself from the event I knew he was attending. I ducked into a nearby restaurant and chose a quiet table where I could do some work. Unbelievably, he came in with a friend and sat at an adjoining table on the side facing me. The three of us struck up a conversation, and I discovered one of the most beautiful, warm, compassionate souls I have ever met. This special and unique man is completely genuine, giving, and passionate about living his life to connect with and inspire others. He is so loved by so many people. There's a light that shines from within him that is recognized by thousands of people once they choose to see the best and most beautiful.

So we often form wrong impressions of others. The key to reversing our misinterpretations is to keep moving forward. Make the choice to be open and brave enough to *risk* letting yourself see and encourage the best in others. This might challenge your innate beliefs, beliefs that have protected you and kept you comfortable. But with this seeking, you might discover the real, genuine human in all their flaws and imperfections—and you might find that beautiful as well, with no changes needed. Every person is entirely special and perfect in their own way, but you have to want and choose to see them that way.

Why should you make this effort to see the best in people? Because people who are treated like they are wonderful, good, and beautiful will come to believe it and become it.

What do you do with those people who are behaving badly? I honestly do not believe that there is anyone who gets up in the morning and says to themselves, "I just want to go out there and be the worst person (or do the worst job) I can today." I think each of us wants to do well and be successful. We want people in our lives to see past our shortcomings or differences, assume that we mean the best, and connect with us in a way that makes that happen. If we mess up today, we want to try again fresh tomorrow, unburdened by the assumption that it will happen again.

If you can do that with the people around you, you'll be building positive relationships and trust. Understanding your biases and recognizing the limitations of your daily impressions will help you engage in ways that make you and everyone around you more successful.

We're different people every day. Try very hard to look at people with fresh eyes. Avoid forming an opinion about them based on something that happened yesterday, on what they look like today, or what someone else may have reported to you. This isn't easy, and we have to be prepared to continually remind ourselves that every day is a new day, we have to question beliefs formed from past information.

Working to make yourself and the people around you better is compassion in action, and it can achieve results in amazing ways!

Exercises for Day 10

· Think about someone you may have made negative judgments about or may have labeled in a way that's not entirely accurate. Is there anything you might be missing? Was it a temporary situation that needs to be put aside and moved past?

· Stretch exercise: Seek out someone you have a negative opinion about based on your assumptions or their appearance. (It requires great honesty on your part to admit your bias.) See if you can get to know them a little better; find something good, beautiful, and special in them.

————————— **Reflections** —————————

1. Describe at least one instance from today when you learned something new and good about someone because you chose to.

2. How did you feel?

3. What is a possible positive result from this instance?

11.

Feel Compassion in the Moment

"Don't wait for extraordinary opportunities.
Seize common occasions and make them great.
Weak men wait for opportunities; strong men make them."

—ORISON SWETT MARDEN

When my daughter Denae was thirteen years old, she was diagnosed with osteosarcoma, a cancer of the bone. Her treatment required a long, grueling course of action that began with surgery to remove the tumor and was followed by several months of in-patient chemotherapy infusions, proton radiation, and several months more of chemo.

She came to deeply dread the long four-hour car rides back and forth to San Francisco and the weekly hospital admits that took place over twelve months. She hated the big, sterile, clinically focused hospitals and what she felt was impersonal care given by highly trained interns. To her, it seemed like she was just another case or room number.

In the midst of all of that anonymity, one person recognized and seized an unexpected opportunity to act with compassion, in the moment. His simple gesture had a profound impact. It succeeded in making my daughter feel special.

On one trip, we had stopped at a red light in front of the building. A group of people began crossing the street in front of us, and we saw within the group one of Denae's doctors. He was the orthopedic half of the international surgical team that had removed the tumor from her spine many months prior. In our pre-op meetings, he had taken a special interest in my daughter because she was a redhead, and he had three redheaded girls!

This world-renowned surgeon glanced over, and our eyes met. He looked at me, then at my daughter in the passenger seat, then back to me. Then he did something we almost couldn't believe. He stepped out of the crosswalk, came around to the passenger side of the car, and, leaning through the open window, he gave Denae a big, long hug. Then he smiled, waved, and was gone.

Denae looked at me and said, "He knows who I am." I could clearly see the joy in her eyes. She felt recognized, real, human.

Thinking about it later, I realized how seizing an opportunity, no matter how unexpected or untimely, can make all the difference in the world to someone else. This man acted on impulse when he stepped over to gift my daughter with that wonderful hug. He could not have seen that chance meeting coming. He could just as easily have looked away from us or simply waved. We would have thought no less of him if he had little or no reaction. He's a busy surgeon. But he did take action. Though it's been twenty years, I've never forgotten that instantaneous, genuine kindness.

We often make all sorts of detailed plans and design strategies for how we're going to demonstrate our caring for the people around us, including patients, coworkers, and staff. In addition to the cards, phone calls, and other pre-determined "stuff," maybe we could pay a little more attention to the impromptu opportunities we encounter and be brave enough to take the initiative to take action. Most of these chances to act are one-of-a-kind and will never happen again in the same way.

Exercises for Day 11

- Be especially aware of those around you, in person and on the phone. Everywhere.

continued

· Note and understand how your smile, word, touch, and mere presence matters. Very much. Give your presence and your attention when you see the opportunity.

--- **Reflections** ---

1. What opportunities did I notice today? How did I respond?

2. How do I feel about the result for me and for the other person?

3. How would I have handled things differently, if at all? Do I wish I had a chance for a do-over? Will I have a chance?

12.

Make Eye Contact
with Meaning

"Let my soul smile through my heart, and let my heart
smile through my eyes . . . that I may scatter
Thy smile in sad hearts freely, everywhere."

—PARAMAHANSA YOGANANDA

As one of our five senses, sight plays a big role in how we learn
about our environment and gather information. Partly through
our vision, we become aware of the objects and scenery surrounding us. Looking at objects and scenery is a passive activity, a one-
way transaction. For instance, if I see a table, it doesn't see me
back. There's no exchange taking place. When we interact with
other people, however, the eyes become a key player in how we
understand and communicate with each other.

Eyes are an enormous factor in how living things are able to express themselves and their feelings. The slightest adjustment of a brow up or down, the narrowing of the eyelids, a crinkle formed in a corner—all these and thousands of other tiny nuances convey a myriad of slightly different messages. The range of emotions that can be sent via the eyes and their immediate area are uncountable. Even if everything on a person's face were covered except the eyes, we would still be able to read meaning in them.

Leadership training, patient care, and even basic customer service education recognizes just how important eye contact is when working with people we serve. "Smile and make eye contact" is a familiar phrase to most of us. Looking at someone directly with a smile is encouraged as a behavior that projects honesty and compassion in a variety of care settings.

When people fail to make eye contact you probably don't feel like you have their attention, even if the rest of their body and their words say you do. Consider how you feel when a salesperson is facing you, head forward, smiling but with their eyes looking elsewhere as they say, "Good morning! How can I help you?" You feel disregarded, unimportant. In cases where you suspect that eye contact is being avoided deliberately you might even suspect deceit, or at the very least a less-than-honest exchange.

Making eye contact is only the beginning of our communication. Communication must be accompanied by compassion to result in connection. Remember our formula:

COMMUNICATION + COMPASSION = CONNECTION

Communication alone doesn't equal connection. Compassion without communicating it isn't connection. We have to combine the two actions to consciously make a connection. Connections are the building blocks of relationships.

To show compassion, you need to use all your available senses, in the moment, and be open and fully engaged in expressing honest intentions and emotions. Looking directly at someone throughout a communication and changing your eye expression to show that you're listening and understanding what's being said is brave. One of the most important ways you can signal to another person that you're both open and engaged is through your eyes.

To try this out, imagine that you're listening to a child tell a story. It might be a sad, happy, or exciting story, and you would probably be exaggerating the reactions of your eyes to show that you are listening and following along. Visualize this conversation, where you're communicating support with your eyes and reacting while the child fully expresses what they're trying to say. If only we could offer such acceptance and encouragement with adults, it might look like this:

- You approach the interaction with a relaxed, soft expression and gaze.

- You look out with gentleness, invitation, and expectation. Your eyes are welcoming.

- When you share glances, you are direct but not piercing. You give encouragement, concern, understanding, and support using your eyes.

Try it in the mirror. Like most of the chapters in this book, just reading about and understanding the activity isn't going to produce change or growth.

The more you practice this the more you'll form genuine relationships that are built on trust. These are the foundation for satisfying our human needs, whether at home or at work: trust, understanding, being heard, being seen, and acknowledgment.

We need to use our growing engagement skills to enhance connections with our staff, coworkers, or patients. To be compassionate, we must put more effort into seeing eye-to-eye and understanding others.

Communicating your caring, openness, and approachability through expressive eyes is a profound way to foster loving, healthy cultures around you.

Exercises for Day 12

- Use the tips in this chapter to change the way you use your eyes today. This is especially easy if you have a child available to share a story with you. If not, practice with someone you trust. Ask them what your eyes are saying as you try different expressions.

- Close your eyes in front of a mirror. Feel each of these emotions: anger, frustration, welcome, warmth, love, curiosity, and apathy. As you take on each one, or others that you think of, open your eyes and look. Do you see that emotion in your eyes?

· Talk to a trusted friend about the expressions in your eyes. Do you both agree on what you were "saying"?

· Make notes as you go through the day and take a few moments to reflect on them tonight.

Reflections

1. How much do you think your eyes express what you're feeling? How open and friendly is your gaze? Would you feel comfortable talking to you?

2. How valuable was this exercise? What would you like to change or work on with regard to what you are communicating with your eyes?

13.

Smile with the Heart

"A warm smile is the universal language of kindness."

—WILLIAM ARTHUR WARD

The smile is a powerful tool in our quest toward more genuine communication and deeper connections. The simple smile can reach out across multiple barriers of language and cultures. It sends out a positive message of greeting and acceptance.

I remember once driving into an unfamiliar neighborhood in a large metropolitan city. I felt alone as I passed dozens of people on the sidewalks and in vehicles all around me. I had been driving for hours that day, with no conversation and no human contact except for the radio. I felt very removed, anonymous, tiny, and unimportant.

While waiting at a red light, I watched a young man as he stepped off a city bus. It looked like he was getting off work or maybe school. It seemed from his relaxed attitude that it was the end of his day. Our eyes met. At first I was a little embarrassed, and I almost looked away, but with an effort I didn't. Instead I lifted my hand in a quick little wave hello. He smiled. I smiled back. I drove off and my mood felt lighter, the city felt brighter, and I didn't feel quite so alone.

The smile can transcend space in a crowded room, on a busy highway, or in places where it's too loud to talk. If you smile at a person and the person smiles back, you both share a warm, good experience. A smile can be an engagement between two people when words aren't possible.

The smile is a central player in the interactions of our daily lives. It affects how we perceive others and how we are perceived by them. If we're not smiling at anyone, and we just naturally smile as a way of conducting ourselves, it tells other people a lot about us.

William Hazlitt said, "A gentle word, a kind look, a good-natured smile can work wonders and accomplish miracles." Any human interaction can be made better, even happier, with a good-natured smile. Smiles enhance understanding between two people. Besides happy smiles there are quizzical smiles, sarcastic smiles, condescending smiles, fake smiles, sad smiles, lonely smiles, and smiles of surrender. A smile can communicate a wide range of emotions and messages. But it is communication, and communication must take place to pave the way to compassion.

Our learning throughout the book is based on awareness and bravery. Smiles require bravery. We might send out a smile, and it might be rejected. But isn't it a wonderful feeling when we get a smile back?

Exercises for Day 13

Do at least two of these four practices:

· Today, think about how you express yourself and impact other people through your smiles. You're going to begin to see how important your smile is. Sometimes a smile is more important than what is said.

Specifically, be attentive to these three things:

· when you smile,

· how you smile, and

· why you smile.

Be brave! Make eye contact *and* share a smile with someone you don't know. Hold your smile for a second longer than you normally would.

· Try sharing a *gentle* smile with at least one person.

· Use different types of smiles. Research different smiles on the internet—you'll be surprised to find as many as fifty smiles.

————————— **Reflections** —————————

1. Today I learned that according to my research there are
   _____ types of smiles.

2. My big, brave smiling moment today came when I shared a gentle
   smile with _____, and it felt _____.

14.

Know That Teams
Must Understand
Before They Can Work

"Teamwork is the ability to work together toward a common vision.
The ability to direct individual accomplishments
toward organizational objectives. It is the fuel that allows
common people to attain uncommon results."

—ANDREW CARNEGIE

We were introducing a newly designed performance evaluation tool to our staff in all the nursing units. The previous off-the-shelf form, which had been used for many years, reflected purely individual performance. We had begun the transition to the team concept by carrying out team-building exercises with staff in different disciplines, including certified nursing assistants, licensed practical nurses, registered nurses, housekeepers, and dietary aides. The pioneering tool was divided into three sections: individual assessment vs. position goals/competencies (40 percent), team goals/metrics (30 percent), and department objectives (30 percent). The purpose was to connect the dots between individual job descriptions, unit metrics, and the strategic plans and objectives that drive the organization as a whole.

Humans are hardwired for cooperation and belonging. From our earliest days, living and working in a pack enhanced our probability of surviving and thriving.

Even today, we are more likely to be successful and happy in life, as well as able to overcome its challenges, if we embrace and are embraced within a community. This means pooling our talents and resources to achieve shared goals. It also means coexisting alongside one another, even when we're striving to reach goals that are *individual*.

Many people think they are better, more effective even, when they act purely for their own benefit.

These are people whose mottos are phrases such as "Every man for himself," "It's a dog-eat-dog world," and "Each to his own." They may believe that survival of the fittest means that the strongest member of a species is the one that lasts and thrives. Anyone who thinks that way should take a few moments today to consider that this survival truism also applies to the fittest *group*, and thus the individuals within that group.

Continuing on with the story about the new performance appraisal tool, to our disappointment, the form went out to loud complaints from some of the nursing staff. They rebelled at the idea that their review, and any possible pay increase, would be dependent on someone else, on something that they thought was outside of their control or ability to influence.

This individualistic thinking is a major and ongoing issue in nursing. Nurses, sadly, have a reputation for "eating their young" and forming "mean girls" clubs. New staff, especially those who don't quickly conform to the "way we do things around here," can be viewed as inconvenient, unwanted, and disruptive. Staff who try to stand up for themselves, those who decide to speak up about this treatment, are more severely ostracized. In my experience, there is often a philosophy that one nurse summed up in her statement about teamwork: "I come in here. I do my job. Alone. I don't want to work with anyone else. I don't want to be part of a team."

My daughter experienced this during her sonography clinicals in a city hospital. The person training her said, "I don't know why they gave you to me. I don't want to train you, and I don't have the time. I can't get my work done with you here."

This is truly tragic for healthcare. There is a constant turnover of staff in challenging markets where there may not be enough quality candidates to begin with. The rotating door results in a need for almost continuous onboarding and training. This in turn puts increased demand on the seasoned nurses and causes burnout. Burnout causes increased call-outs, staff "working short," and resignations. And the cycle goes on.

Working in nursing demands that we welcome and use the talents of every single person. Think of a football team. Each player has their part to play, and they are skilled and practiced in what they do. At the same time, each player has to know and be able to rely on the gifts of other players to reach the goal post. There cannot be a team of all quarterbacks or kickers, and it would be impossible for one player to make it down the field to score against an opposing group that *is* acting as a team and using their combined abilities.

Again, our revised performance evaluation showcased the advantages of team members sharing their talents to work toward common goals. With time, and an adjusting of the annual reviews to a common date,[1] we saw results reflected in not only our metrics but also in everyday stories: staff eating and taking breaks together in different groups, more problem-solving efforts in regular meetings, decreased absenteeism, staff helping each other on the floor and behind the doors, and one staffer even shared with me that she believed that her patient was a team member. Ongoing discussion of progress and successes became a more common occurrence among employees and between employees and their supervisors.

---

1   We adjusted 100 percent of the staff to a common review date so they would all be working toward the same goals and objectives on the same calendar timetable.

In business and leadership, a common, clear goal that is loudly and publicly proclaimed is a must. The objectives that support reaching that goal must be achievable and real for every member of the team. Each member must be able to not only envision but truly feel how their effort, combined with the efforts of others, will result in tangible benefits to all. The goal of healthcare, for example, is to provide quality care to the population with which we work. To be most effective, each staff member must be able to see how we impact the quality of care so that we can stay focused. We also must be clear about who we need to partner with, and we have to learn how to work together.

Lastly, each of us has to feel like we have the ability to truly impact the ultimate achievement of individual or team goals. We have to be patient, because understanding and seeing this picture can take time.

Today is the beginning of your awareness of the big picture that forms if each of us is willing to have compassion for the other, to understand them, and to work successfully together.

Exercises for Day 14

- Consider carefully today how what you do fits in to the overall organization and its goals.
- At the end of the day you should be able to write about at least one example of how your efforts contribute to your organization as a whole.

continued

- Next describe at least one way in which you feel your efforts are *not* contributing to the big picture.

———————————— **Reflections** ————————————

1. Hopefully you identified and observed a specific activity today and how it fits into the big picture of your company. What was it? Is it individual to you, or is it a team goal?

2. How much influence do you think you have in reaching the objective? Do you have the span of control needed?

3. How do you feel compassion relates to achieving objectives with and through your teammates? Or, if you're a leader, how does compassion relate to working together with the teams around you?

Act

We deliberately propel forward to take
action, to have an effect on our
environment. We move.

We become increasingly adept at creating
motion by practicing small, specific behaviors.
We repeat them until they start to become habits. We then build on these new foundations.

We lean beyond reaction; we are proactive.

We drive change.

15.

Model Compassion to Others

"We learn by example and by direct experience because
there are real limits to the adequacy of verbal instruction."

—MALCOLM GLADWELL

Health-care organizations, like most companies, spend millions
of dollars every year on training and staff education. When there's
a well-crafted approach to staff development, this education takes
a wide variety of forms and formats, from formal orientation and
onboarding of new hires to in-servicing for new products, policies, and protocols, and attendance at conferences, enrollment in
college courses, and mentoring and buddy-type programs.

For healthcare, the bulk of the training provided is required by
regulation and is heavily monitored by outside agencies as a condition of licensing. Even in good companies with the best intentions these trainings sometimes become an exercise of checking

off boxes on government lists. The value of the initial investments can be diminished when there is a lack of follow-up or a lack of continuation of the learning relationship.

In addition to the documented millions budgeted and spent, money is lost when training is absent or has been ineffective. These dollars are hard to capture. Here are some examples:

- Spending $1,000 for two weeks of scheduled training for a new hire but failing to provide more dollars for additional support as the new employee transitions into the workforce
- Not studying why and how a costly training effort with a current employee failed, so that possible remedies can be considered rather than losing the value of the training or letting the employee go
- Money lost in productivity and errors from untrained employees who stay
- Loss of morale when team-building is absent
- Decline in consumer satisfaction, employee engagement, quality scores and outcomes, and other measurables due to lessened confidence in the competence of staff

Overall the impact is staggering. So what do we do? If we had more resources, we might do what all great organizations strive to do: reach past the required training to invest in organizational efficiencies, competency confirmation, cross-departmental work, individual growth projects, and projects affecting all cultural and communication areas.

Let's assume, though, that we are limited in terms of additional dollars or hours for training and staff development. This is a frequent response to any suggestion of new initiatives. What can we do to make the best of the money and time we put into training and growing our people?

Let's talk about a free and invaluable tool called modeling. When someone acts or takes action, they're modeling a behavior or activity. Modeling is a very powerful teaching method. People often learn more about us from what we do than from what we say. So it's imperative that we pay attention to what we're telling them.

I observed a very clear example of people saying one thing and modeling another a few days ago, when I was having breakfast at Denny's. Two women were at an adjoining booth with an infant and a toddler. Both of them, apparently mother and grandmother, were teaching good manners to a darling little girl by having her use "please" and "thank you" as she interacted with them during breakfast. "Pancake" and a pointed finger was changed to "Pancake, please." As I watched the two women conversing and making requests of the young waiter, I noticed that they weren't using please or thank you with him. I wondered if the little girl was paying attention. She kept close watch on her mother and grandmother and the waiter as he fetched ketchup, more napkins, and coffee refills. It was obviously lost on them that they weren't doing what they were telling her to do.

This story shows how easily we can send conflicting messages despite our best intentions.

Before we get to your exercise for today, please consider and choose to agree that one of the most effective, lasting, and low-cost methods we can use for teaching the people around us, the people who may work for us, and the people we serve and care for is modeling. Modeling basically works when a subject is watched doing or acting or being in a way that is correct and acceptable and then another subject copies (mimics) what they've seen so that they can repeat the desired behavior.

Almost everything about us, everywhere we go, is being continually observed. What we do, how we move, what we say, and how we say it. No matter what we try to put forth about who we are, and what is right and what is important to us, others will most often look to our actions to determine what is true and real.

In the world of work, regardless of what has been shared as the "desired" behavior or culture, the new employee who's trying to fit in or the current employee who wants to excel and move up will take note of what the successful "other" models. The successful other could be a nurse who is popular or has longevity, a coworker who is being promoted or recognized publicly, or someone who has been chosen as a leader, such as a manager or administrator.

New hires may receive formal training on policies, protocols, and practices, and may see literature on company culture and expectations. But some of the most meaningful education takes place after the training when they observe what people actually say and do.

We all strive to portray ourselves to the world in a specific way, the way in which we'd like to be viewed. I want to be seen as caring, competent, trustworthy, and a little brave, and I want to leave having made a difference in this world. If this rings a bell with you, we both need to realize that it's not about what we say we want or who we say we are or what we tell others to do in our daily interactions. It's more important that we actually practice how we would like to be viewed. For example, we should strive to model compassion, moment by moment, action by action, if we want to be viewed as a compassionate person. If you strive to be viewed as compassionate, you should show people what it looks like so they can mimic it, experience the results, and become intentionally compassionate themselves.

Exercises for Day 15

Thoughtfully consider your actions. How much difference is there between what you are telling others to say and do vs. what you actively model in your words and actions? How do your behaviors align with company culture?

- As you work with those around you, your coworkers, those who look up to you as an authority, and even your patients or residents, what do your actions say about you?

- Are you modeling compassion in your actions, words, and tone of voice? How are you modeling the compassion that you

continued

expect to see in others? If you're not, what could you have done to handle things differently?

· Stretch exercise: Consider what is being modeled to you by your peers and leaders.

Reflections

1. Who did you observe exercising compassion today? How did it affect you? Can you mimic it?

2. How can formal and informal leaders line their words up with their actions when it comes to compassion?

3. What type of modeling, or steps, do you think can "teach" compassion in the workplace? How would you help the best and most caring nurses share what they know and help others act more compassionately?

16.

Choose Personal Interaction over Technology Whenever Possible

"We get addicted to the rush at work, or to the endless flow of
the online world, and your life changes. Attention spans go down,
patience decreases, essential tasks are left undone,
and most of all, our humanity starts to fade away."

—SETH GODIN

My first real job was in 1979. I worked for the state of
Nevada as a public service intern. This meant that I basically did all kinds of reports, studies, memos, and odd
assignments—the work that was important enough to
get done but not so earth-shaking that an intern couldn't

do it. My office consisted of three cubicle walls, a phone, yellow legal pads, pens, a desk calculator, a stapler, and staples. The only keyboard in sight was a shared IBM Selectric typewriter on a rolling stand. When people needed to communicate they either called each other on the telephone or they met face to face.

Fast forward to today. My most recent in-office work setting looked very different. Walking through an office suite, I'd see people staring into computer screens, typing away to share information, say hello, and communicate with their teams. On their desk was a cellphone, which got a glance every few minutes throughout the day. Face-to-face meetings happened, but it seemed that people were constantly communicating through technology—even during their face-to-face meetings. I'd often hear someone in the hall greet a coworker with, "Did you get my email?"

Recently I passed a bus stop on a beautiful spring morning in Washington, D.C., and it struck me that there were six people standing within feet of each other, each staring and "engaging" on their cell phone with someone in another place. Hopefully they were planning a future get-together!

Although technology such as email and texting may help us communicate with other people on the fly, I believe its highest value might be in helping us plan to meet in person and catch up on ideas we want to discuss or share. What we hopefully are seeking in email and text messages is to arrange a true connection.

Technology is useful when we need to get a consistent, repetitive message out to a large number of people at once. Or if we have to share plans that include lots of details, numbers, or other types of data, whether in-house or across geographic areas and companies.

Managers and leaders who want to actually have real relationships and show others the optimal way to do that must step a-w-a-y from technology, which is merely a tool, and interact in person. This also means leaving your cell phone at your desk. I feel the need to say this because I have seen leaders leave their office only to walk down the halls with—you guessed it—their eyes glued to their cell phone.

Interestingly, I read recently that younger managers and those hoping to be managers actually do not support teleworking for their company's top executives. It seems that they want these role models physically in the office where they can have personal contact and facetime, which they feel contributes much more to their success than virtual encounters. This is very insightful on their part and reinforces my point that in person trumps technology.

When it comes to relationships, email and autobots might be better than nothing, but it may be best to reserve them as a last resort. When email is used to express opinions and feelings, it can lead to very serious misunderstandings. (I say this from decades of human resources experience!) How often have we found that we need to circle back to clarify, give more information, or calm down an irate person who misinterpreted what was said? What might have been a "missed" communication has now become a "miscommunication." There's no efficiency there.

You may believe you need all the information you are sent, but we're being overloaded with *mountains* of information. And if you receive numerous messages all at once, you can't possibly process them effectively. And you don't need to! What you need to do is take control and be thoughtful about what data you can use and seek it out.

The technology that's been developed in the past forty years is meant to enhance our ability to communicate by streamlining our documentation and making it easier to keep in touch, right? So are we better connected? Do we reach out and touch each other in meaningful ways with this "extra" time we have?

In medicine specifically, we have moved to electronic medical records, computer screens for CNA charting ease, portable tablets used by providers during patient visits, and more. This may have been partially intended to allow more personal, quality time with the patient; in reality that personal touch can be lost in a sea of detail.

Here's a personal example:

My thirteen-year-old daughter was being treated for bone cancer at one of the best teaching hospitals in the country, one that specializes in pediatric oncology. The hospital was very organized, professional, and knowledgeable, but it was also unfortunately cold and institutional in its care approach. The doctors made their daily rounds with clipboards in hand, discussing vital signs, cancer staging numbers, and chemotherapy regimen specifics. There was little, if any, doctor-to-patient eye contact, and no conversation with us. We were surprised when one morning a physician resident in training spoke directly to the little bald-headed girl lying in the bed. We were thrilled to think that he might be seeing past all the data in her chart. But that happiness changed to disappointment when he leaned over, looked in her eyes, and said, "How are you today, young man?" She was devastated. With all the information available he failed to notice something very special and important to her, her gender. The experience tainted her view of the hospital and made an extremely aggressive course of treatment even harder to bear. (It was the spontaneous act of compassion by the surgeon in the crosswalk, in my previous story, that helped turn this around. There is almost always an opportunity to make a difference.)

Consider that the true role of a leader is not fulfilled in front of a computer screen or from behind a desk or a closed office door. It comes from interacting as personally as we can, in every situation, every day.

Think of it this way: When you are in your office, you are probably doing. When you are participating alongside the people in their work lives, you are being—being a leader.

The moral is not to let the information and data overwhelm us or cloud our vision of what is right in front of us. See the individual behind the numbers. Get what we need, then step away from the screen! Be there to really engage with the people and happenings around us, instead of just reading about them.

Exercises for Day 16

- Walk around today, and leave your cell phone in your office. Step away from your desk, desktop, laptop, voicemail, social networks, and out into the reality of the world that is being played out where you work.

- Go out there with wide open ears and eyes, a bunch of curiosity, and as little fear as possible. It may feel strange. You might not feel like you're "doing" anything, but go with it. If you get the sense that people are wondering what you are up to, take it as a sure sign that you really need to do this more often. If you're really, really uncomfortable having no valid agenda, then it's okay to drop off a note to someone down the hall or look for someone so that you can ask them a question. The note or question might be something you would normally email or call for, but delivering or asking in person is a great excuse to go out and about. But don't make a beeline to your destination and buzz right back. Enjoy the journey. Take time to jot some notes tonight.

- And then do it again, for a little longer, tomorrow. I promise it gets better.

Reflections

1. Be honest. How long did you spend outside of your office today?

2. Write down something good that happened today. (Sometimes it takes a while for it to come back around. If that happens you can come back and add it later.)

3. List any vital, crucial, undelayable phone call, text, or email that you missed because you weren't in front of a screen.

4. If there were any, how did you manage the situation?

17.

Move Forward by Slowing Down

"Clarity and decisiveness come from the willingness to slow down, to listen to and look at what's happening."

—PEMA CHÖDRÖN

Slowing down is one of the top things I advise leaders to do if they want to be more effective, get more done, and have better relationships with their teams. Although it doesn't seem logical, to move ahead you have to slow down.

I recently conducted an exit interview with an employee named Stephanie. We came to a question on the survey about Stephanie's relationship with her supervisor, asking her to rate this relationship on a scale from "Highly Satisfied" to "Highly Dissatisfied." Stephanie told me that she didn't know how to answer the question, because she didn't have a relationship with her supervisor. In fact, she wasn't even clear who her supervisor was.

Stephanie's shift is one of the challenges of many 24/7 work environments. She worked the 7 p.m.–3 a.m. shift, and she had very little, if any, interaction with her teammates or the team leaders. This makes it hard for the worker to have a sense of belonging and is challenging for the supervisors.

But what truly struck me was when Stephanie said that when she did chance to see her managers, it seemed like "they were all rushing around and all into their business. I never felt like I should bother them or interrupt them." She had worked for the company for almost a year with little feedback, except for emails correcting errors she'd made on the job. (Remember that we talked about emails as poor communication? They are especially poor choices for addressing work performance issues.)

I've known managers like the one Stephanie described. They have an energy around them that sends the message that they are involved in an extremely important task and should not be stopped. While multitasking may be good in some circumstances, they do it to a fault, and to the detriment of their work—no one thing is done as well as it may have been, given their full attention. They carry this energy in a way that is a shield against being approached by people who may need them. Knowingly or not, they distance themselves from people they are there to serve, people who *are* the business at hand. (If only I had a nickel for every time a manager has said, "I could get so much more done if I didn't have all these people interruptions." Those managers are not leaders.)

Sometimes we can get caught up in the doing of our work and lose sight of the importance of being there for those we lead and supervise. While there are times when we are actually too busy with another task that takes priority in the moment, it's just as important to make time for people, to ensure that they feel comfortable coming to us with their concerns, questions, ideas, or whatever it is.

During the course of our discussions, I asked Stephanie if I could talk with her team and her supervisor, and if we could make it better would she be willing to reconsider leaving. She said yes, and we all met to share her thoughts, feelings, and suggestions as well as discuss options workable for the entire group. I stepped out as they were wrapping up on their own. Ultimately, she did stay, which was wonderful because she was a conscientious, caring employee, and it was a very difficult shift to fill. New communication strategies were planned, including regular staff meetings, ongoing logs, and clarified security protocols.

Achievers, keep in mind that just because you're moving faster doesn't mean that you're getting more done. Doing is not always the true measure of effectiveness, although it is one factor in competence. The ultimate accomplishment of a leader is the strength of their influence, how their being impacts and drives others.

Exercises for Day 17

Slow. Down.

- No matter how busy you are, strive to avoid pushing people away who might really need you. Save your stressed,

continued

busy-looking self for real emergencies. Monitor yourself
throughout the day. Look in a mirror if it helps!

- If you need a visual, picture yourself as a duck floating on a
  lake. Although underneath your (duck) feet are frantically
  paddling back and forth to propel you through the water, on
  the surface you appear serene, quiet, calm, almost motionless.

- Breathe! Look up! Smile first!

- Pay attention to how much more connected you feel with the
  people and things that surround you.

Reflections

1. How did you DO today at "being"?

2. Describe a specific something good that happened today because
   you slowed down.

18.

Be Generous
with Offers to Help

"Once you've done the mental work, there comes a point you have to
throw yourself into action and put your heart on the line."

—PHIL JACKSON

As with the "slow down to speed up" advice, being generous
with offers to help might seem counterproductive. Most of us
are short on time and sometimes short on people. We're all-
around short, busy, and tired. How can we possibly offer more
help? Bear with me as I take you back to my time at Washoe
Health System, now RENOWN.

It was time to review the most recent patient satisfaction
scores for the large hospital. An important rating related directly
to patient experience—"staff takes time to care for my needs"—
had taken a dive from the prior year. Reorganization had placed

a new set of pressures on our staff. "How can we make things less painful for our people and less obvious to the patients?" our Customer Satisfaction Team asked.

Among the solutions we offered was to begin closing patient/customer encounters with the question, "Is there anything else that I can do for you while I'm here?" The staff initially resisted, concerned that they wouldn't be able to offer more time and more services when clearly they were already stretched to capacity. But we moved forward with a "let's try it" attitude. The results were astonishing.

Most of the customers when asked replied, "No, there is nothing else. Thank you!" The encounter felt complete and ended on a positive note. Another small number, maybe 15 to 20 percent, replied with an additional request, which was usually simple, and quickly and easily met, such as, "Can you fluff my pillow?" or "Could you please get me a drink?" This need would have ultimately required attention anyway, and it possibly would have been a more urgent and inconvenient interruption later. Some issues needed follow-up research of course, but these were started sooner rather than later because of the staff's proactive questioning.

The staff had worried about facing a larger burden, but the actual results showed the opposite. Later, they self-reported feeling more organized and less stressed, with a higher level of job and task satisfaction. They also shared that they felt more immediate appreciation for their efforts.

The patients and other customers also described a higher

level of satisfaction with the services and the care they received. The next survey showed better ratings for their perceptions of both staff skills and the quality of caring.

Exercises for Day 18

· No matter when or how another person comes to seek your attention today, practice greeting them with a smile and a sincere hello.

· At the end of meetings, try to ask each time, "Is there anything else I can do for you?" or "While I'm here, is there anything else I can do?" (Tip: I've learned always to carry a pen and paper for notetaking.)

You may be surprised at the immediate results of using these little phrases, and you might also see a look of pleasant surprise from the person. In any case, I believe you'll see an increase in confidence in your competence from the people you and your teams serve, and that's the best surprise.

Reflections

1. What opportunities did you have to try out the two phrases today?

2. What requests did people have of you that you weren't able to fulfill?

3. What was the reaction of people when you asked the questions?

4. How likely are you to use these questions tomorrow?

19.

Know That Compassion and Accountability Go Hand-in-Hand

"Part of being a compassionate boss is clearly outlining what you
expect in terms of behavior, results, and impact. When people
don't meet our expectations, it's all too easy to jump to conclusions.
Compassion is rooted in a profound respect for others and reflects an
unfailing commitment to uphold the dignity of people."

—NIKI LEONDAKIS (CEO EQUINOX FITNESS CLUBS,
FORMER COO KIMPTON HOTELS)

Some statements you might hear when you bring compassion
and business into the same sentence are:

"There is no place for compassion in business."

"Business isn't personal. People shouldn't bring their feelings and emotions in to work."

"We're here to produce. I'm responsible for making that happen."

"I take responsibility and so should my team and my coworkers. I don't have time for worrying about what's going on with them."

"It's not my business."

"You shouldn't wear your heart on your sleeve."

I have personally heard every one of these statements, and many more, at work and in talking about this book project.

Whether we choose to recognize it or not, feelings affect every worker, every day. Work is personal. Feelings are real. Unfortunately, we're asked in management to leave our feelings at home. We ask our staff to do the same. We've become desensitized and, yes, when it comes to our role as leaders to direct optimal work performance, we are afraid to approach that line where compassion and caring meet accountability and responsibility. But the success of our employees and the company depends on our willingness to act in caring ways, to model the same behaviors with our staff that we would expect to see with, for example, our residents, patients, or customers. So what do we do?

One of the biggest objections I've heard to being compassionate in the workplace is that there will be a reduction in accountability. In the human resources office, we often are faced with balancing the caring with the facts. Over the years, I have found that daring to act in caring ways yields incredible results in terms of employee relations. Honesty, empathy, and clarity are all forms of compassion. And it seems like managers are afraid to be these things because they might cross the line.

At work we sometimes put up shields to keep ourselves from becoming too involved with other human beings. It's normal. For me it's often because I'm afraid of being taken advantage of, of giving or promising too much, or of being seen as not objective enough. But what if we made a conscious decision to watch our boundaries yet be brave enough to be flexible? What if we were taught to be comfortable with taking caring action while still maintaining control? If we could allow ourselves to be brave enough to get closer to that imaginary line, prepared for the fact that it's a little uncomfortable, we would be on the path to experiencing a connection that results in deeper, more engaged interactions. The risk is worth it don't you think?

There are two keys to successfully walking the line between compassion and accountability, both of which rely on clear communication, mutual understanding, and agreement. And both require forethought and awareness.

One key is to know one's personal and professional boundaries. A little discomfort is all right. Exploring our discomfort helps us grow and deepen the quality of our relationships. But how will we define what is non-negotiable? To define boundaries, all leaders must develop an understanding of themselves and relate that understanding back to their own and the company's core values. As leaders and workers we have to think about and answer these questions:

- What are we willing and able to do?
- What guides our decisions?
- How will we recognize and knowingly make the choice to cross a boundary?
- How will we know and be willing to recognize and honor when another's boundaries are being pushed, when we're insisting on pushing another's comfort line in a painful way?

These questions require a high degree of sensitivity on our parts, something all leaders must have. First, know thyself!

The second key is mutual understanding and agreement regarding the details of the accountability. I have found that holding people accountable to clear expectations is one of the most compassionate actions we can take in business. We cannot hold someone accountable for something they did not know—or in some cases did not know how—to do. That's why communicating clear expectations and quickly addressing small "shortcomings" is so crucial. Ironically, sometimes managers themselves aren't clear about what the expectations are until they are not met.

Approaching accountability discussions with honesty and caring builds trust. When we're assigned responsibility for an employee, it's also part of that responsibility to cultivate a trusting relationship by being appropriately open with and allowing them the same openness.

Listening before judging and taking accountability for any lapse that may have occurred in communication are two actions that bring us closer to meeting our mutual goals. People share more of themselves in companies that are free from a culture of fear, which creates huge opportunities for trust and collaboration.

Exercises for Day 19

Think about an accountability discussion that you might be having today or in the near future.

- Do you have any uneasiness about the conversation? Why or why not?

- Is there more homework you need to do before the meeting? (You might feel uncomfortable, but remember the employee is probably more uncomfortable, possibly even scared. I don't think employees should be scared at work.)

When you have the conversation, please try these tips:

- Strive to do more listening, to try to understand the employee's perspective.

- Pay attention to behavior, what's not being said. Be open to a deeper conversation if it seems needed.

continued

· Pay attention to the end result of the talk. How did you feel? Did you learn something about yourself or the other person?

Remember: For today you're just paying attention and becoming aware. You're getting to know yourself better. You're exploring that line between compassion and accountability.

————————————— **Reflections** —————————————

1. What do you think about combining authority/accountability with compassion/feelings? What objections do you have, or have you heard?

2. How effective are you at communicating expectations consistently and clearly to people with whom you work?

3. Why or why not? How could you improve?

20.

Seek the Sameness over the Differences

"It's never the differences between people that surprise us.
It's the things that, against all odds, we have in common."

—JODI PICOULT

Similarities can pop up in some truly surprising places. Recently I was in line for coffee at a retirement home in Alexandria, Virginia, where I was working, when I heard a resident mention to another man that he had lived in Turkey. I couldn't stop myself from asking where and when he had been there. When he said Ankara, in the early 1970s, I was amazed! I told him that I had lived in Ankara at the same time. He noted with a grin that our ages were very different, but he said that his three children had attended the school on the Balgat military base. With a little figuring, we realized that his twins had been in the seventh grade with me, and I remembered them. As luck would have it, I still had my junior high yearbook. A few days later I brought it in to work. I showed him that my picture and his children's pictures were on the same page. It astonished us both that we had made an unexpected connection. Through coincidence we discovered something totally and completely obscure that the two of us had in common where before there was nothing![1]

And that's what draws us together. It's in our nature as humans to seek safety and comfort in familiarity. Because of this we consciously or subconsciously gravitate toward people and groups with whom we feel we have something in common. The most obvious commonalities are physical characteristics: age, race, gender, etc., but some are more hidden and need further exploration to be revealed. These could be things about our past, background, experiences, or interests that are shared by someone else.

We will only have the potential to find the deeper core commonalities that transcend our differences if we intentionally take the time to listen, connect, and share with other people. When we operate in a world of assumptions and preconceptions, and maybe false beliefs based on what we see on the outside, or what we think we already know, we miss out on so many chances to discover something new. That stranger on the bus may also love jazz music. The person in line in the grocery store might live two

---

1   As a side note, that opening actually prompted him to come to me with an issue he was reluctant to bring up with other staff members.

doors down or have the same kind of dog or cat. Our coworker may have been raised in the same area we were.

My story of the resident whose children I had gone to school with is just one tiny example, but think about how we pass by one another at our jobs. We are so physically close, yet there is so much unknown between us. There is so much distance between what we know (very little) and what we don't know (lots and lots). At work, people segregate themselves into groups based on obvious factors like job title or function, skill level, language, country of origin, religion, or known personal interests. We sometimes group ourselves by the "sameness" of our differences. If we don't take the time to dig deeper we might really be missing out on a connection, thinking that we share nothing in common with people around us, the people we work for, or the people who work for us. But we do!

We have to be willing to see beyond the differences and be curious about the person. We have to remember that different doesn't mean wrong or bad. Differences aren't something to fear; they simply represent the variety in the human race. Differences aren't something to be hidden; they shouldn't be cause for shame or embarrassment. We are all different. Sometimes it takes effort and imagination to discover where we're the same. We have such a rich tapestry of peoples in our workplaces today, there's no such thing as "one size fits all." We should strive to be open-minded and fair, realizing that equal is not a reality. Equity yes, but not equality. It's a challenge for organizations all around the globe.

But we are given a tremendous advantage working in health-care. We have a common starting point of sameness that many other fields or businesses do not have, and that starting point can help create a culture of inclusion. Workers who are drawn to the healthcare field share a mission. Regardless of the department or discipline they've chosen, they have a mission to help others. It's our responsibility as leaders to keep that fire lit within them for the duration of their careers.

If we can keep the "sameness" of that drive and purpose chan-neled, there are endless possibilities. We can discover how our shared strengths and unique attributes contribute to the success of the community as a whole. When people are invited and wel-comed in, bringing their whole selves, their similarities and dif-ferences, to the health-care workplace, everyone wins.

This chapter is in the Act section because seeking the simi-larities over the differences won't happen unless you consciously make the effort to explore these commonalities. The more you practice, and the more genuine your curiosity becomes, the more likely it is that you'll find things in common with people you thought were very different from you. Why should you care, you ask? What's in it for me? The more you know about people, the more sameness you find, the more you can build real connections and reach common goals.

Exercises for Day 20

· When you're outside your regular work space, take note of the people around you. When you see someone new, or whom you don't work directly with, greet them and see if you can start a casual conversation.

· Talk to the person next to you. Maybe you're in line, maybe you're in an elevator, maybe you're in a meeting and you're sitting next to someone you usually don't sit next to.

· If it feels too uncomfortable now, or the right situations don't present themselves, don't sweat it! Keep an air of curiosity about the people around you. Be poised to jump in and explore further (like I did when the elderly man mentioned that he'd lived in Turkey).

Reflections

1. What new things in common did you discover with your peers, bosses, strangers, patients, residents, and anyone else around you?

2. This exercise is finished when you can share five new things here:

21.

Know the Numbers
but Learn the Stories

"Stories—individual stories, family stories, national stories—
are what stitch together the disparate elements of human
existence into a coherent whole. We are story animals."

—YANN MARTEL

The scenario seems to present itself way too often. We check the news of the morning, and we hear about a large-scale tragedy like an enormously destructive hurricane, a powerful tsunami, an earthquake, or an airplane crash. The numbers of lives affected are staggeringly high. The early number might be relatively low, in the hundreds, but it could also be in the thousands, and it may rise as the day and days pass.

We're temporarily stunned, and our reaction is one of sadness. If the event is something that could realistically have happened to us we internalize it and experience a sense of fear. We think, "That could have been me," and then we feel relief to again realize it wasn't. (Even if it's a good event, like a lottery win when the ticket was bought near our home, we internalize and relate to it depending on our likelihood of experiencing the same good fortune.) The higher the chances it could have happened to us, the more we empathize or share the feelings surrounding it. Then we count our blessings and move on about our day feeling grateful for our life. We typically haven't felt deep pain or sorrow over the incident despite the magnitude of the number of people affected by the event.

Why is that? We're caring, loving people. How can we know about these huge catastrophes and not feel a real, piercing pain? Have we become desensitized?

No, I don't believe that is the answer. We process the facts—dates, times, numbers—and determine how they may relate to us. We shield ourselves in a way, creating a buffer so we can move forward with the new information.

But later, we learn a story behind just one "number," the ending of one life, the tale of one near miss, the sadness of one lost love, the last day of one child. We feel the deep sorrow, the pain, the compassion toward humanity in its individual form.

Even an accountant will tell you, numbers are always just a part of the story. Working as a manager means monitoring a big, ever-changing picture that's made up of many numbers: ratios, percentages, decimal points, cost per hour or per person, inventory counts, and the list goes on. We need identifiers like employee ID numbers, patient numbers, record numbers, and various methods for tracking data, charting trends, and measuring productivity.

A great leader will always remember that behind many of those numbers is a human being, and that it serves us well to learn the stories of the people. Whether it's an employee who is showing up as a number on a turnover report, or a patient or resident whose fall has been documented, the circumstances keep the caring and humanity alive. From the very basic and routine stuff to life-threatening or end-of-life events, we can't lose sight of the face of this one human being who is peeking out from behind the numbers we view on our screen or paper.

We need to schedule time to consider the dashboard of information we face on a monthly, weekly, daily, or even (ugh) hourly basis. We have to plan, do, and check, and then step out of our office, our buffer, and act. Engage with the people and the stories. This takes strength and courage, because you'll be stepping outside your comfort zone.

As you're out there, you can think about what those numbers—good or not so good—mean. Ask people around you, "What do you think this is telling us?" Involve and interact with the teams described by the data; sometimes they have simple answers you may not have thought of. Learn the stories. Act like a detective to explore options. Use critical thinking to make sense of and complete the picture represented by those numbers. Really live the story of the individual by identifying the sameness either with yourself or with a past case. That is where your experience and expertise kick in for the benefit of the people that you serve!

Exercises for Day 21

- Look at the numbers like you always do. Then pick a number that you're concerned or curious about, maybe something that is notably up or down. Maybe it is a production number, for example, or the number of late reviews, absenteeism rates, supply costs, or call bell usage.

- Reach out in person or by phone to the person who could best explain the story behind that number. Ask them for examples.

- Focus on what you're exploring and addressing, but let yourself become involved with, hear, and feel the individual stories. Make your face part of the big picture by getting closer.

Roll up your sleeves (figuratively or for real). Step out from behind the charts, graphs, and data out into the life of your organization.

Reflection

1. I was able to dig deeper behind a "dashboard" number today. Here's what I learned.

2. What numbers do you look at every day that you need to question or get rid of? If there are numbers you don't use or understand, ask why.

Dare to Care

We become more comfortable with the
uncomfortable, more willing to exist in the
gray, closer to the edges of our boundaries.

We recognize the value of taking the
risk to care.

We see that we're not only communicating,
we are also truly connecting.

22.

Consider Other Viewpoints

"Empathy is about standing in someone else's shoes, feeling with his
or her heart, seeing with his or her eyes. Not only is empathy hard to
outsource and automate, but it makes the world a better place."

—DANIEL H. PINK

When my grandmother moved into a nursing home several years
ago, I had recently relocated across the country, from Nevada to
Virginia. I kept in touch with her via phone calls, and I regularly
talked to the staff for updates on her needs. Although her eyesight was becoming severely impacted by macular degeneration,
my Nanor, as we called her, stayed sharp as a tack. She maintained
the strong personality that went with her fiery red hair, referring
to herself as the immaculate degenerate.

During one of my weekly calls to the marble palace, as my
grandmother called it, the staff told me that she'd begun to

require sedatives because she was having delusions and hallucinations. Because the drugs made her unsteady and had caused a minor fall, she had begun using a wheelchair for the first time. On the phone, she had indeed told me that she was constantly surrounded by small green children, even when she was in bed. They were constantly telling her what to do and where to go, day and night. This caused her even more agitation.

On my next visit, I found Nanor in a wheelchair in a common area. I walked up in front of her and gave her a giant hug. I moved with her to a chair, and we sat eye-to-eye and knee-to-knee, talking up a storm. It was during our talk that a petite young CNA in green scrubs came from behind her, squatted down, and said, "Time for your lunch. We need to go."

Nanor pointed to the aide and exclaimed, "See Dee Dee! See? Green."

Mystery solved. Here was the small green child! I shared this with the charge nurse and a note was added to her care plan, along with a re-evaluation of her medications.

This story tells us how important it is to be sensitive to how life is being perceived through the eyes and feelings of another person. As a health-care human resources professional, my primary role has been to support the people who serve the residents or patients. My understanding of their work is aided by the fact that my first job in long-term care was as a medical social worker. I know what it means to serve an elderly, fragile population. So that I can stay in touch with the core of the health-care mission, I always make an effort to connect with the residents and patients. When I explain that I hire, train, and support employees, I get warm and wonderful responses about the staff. It's often something like, "Where do you find so many nice people to work here?"[1]

Every once in a while though, if the time and place are right, a resident will say, "You do training? Can you please help them be more sensitive to how I feel? I just don't think that people who aren't as old and frail as I am always understand how important it is to be gentle. They forget that I *can't* move faster. And my feelings get hurt when I sense their frustration. I know that they're busy and short-staffed, but I wish they could see through my eyes."

We can learn so much from just being intentionally more sensitive to another person's perceptions and abilities. In the case of the elderly, for example, their bodies are more fragile. Their bones and skin are more susceptible to injury, and they are more susceptible to pain. Their eyes and ears don't work the same way they used to. They need our guidance, sometimes our assistance, and always our unwavering patience.

Although we can't replicate exactly what another person is experiencing, we can attempt to consider their perspective before we choose any action on their behalf. What do they encounter with their five senses? What are they seeing, hearing, and touching? Think things through, anticipate needs, explore options, and always involve them in the discussion. Avoid assumptions and misunderstanding, and foster confidence by being compassionate.

---

1   My answer is that nice people attract nice people.

Exercises for Day 22

· Change your view. Sit alongside a resident or patient. Choose a different seat at a meeting or meal table.

· Catch yourself assuming that you know what another person is feeling or seeing. Ask them:

"How are you feeling today?"

"Will you tell me more about that?"

"Is there anything I can do to make things better, make things easier or more comfortable?"

"Is there anything you need?"

Put yourself in their position and listen closely to each response. You'll feel the trust build.

-------------------- **Reflections** --------------------

1. What did you see differently today?

2. What situations did you encounter around you, or observe, that included an opportunity for someone to show more sensitivity?

3. If you changed seats, what was your experience of a different view?

23.

Understand Emotions
without Taking Them On

"We cannot control what emotions or circumstances we will
experience next, but we can choose how we respond to them."

—GARY ZUKAV

Why is it that one person will get in a small fender-bender, pull
over, exchange insurance information, smile, and go about their
day taking it in stride, while another will get in a small fender
bender, pull over to scream, yell, rant, rave, and cry, exchange
information, and then go home having decided that it was a
totally bad day?

Neither person is nicer or better than the other. One is not a
more highly skilled driver. They were both rear-ended and not at
fault. It's not that one is easygoing and the other is a hothead. It's
simply that they are having different emotional reactions to the

same circumstances based on how they're feeling and their overall experiences that day.

If the exact same thing were to happen tomorrow, they could react entirely differently.

They are *not* their emotions; they are still just them.

None of us are our emotions. We can be angry, sad, afraid, joyful, or frustrated. But that is not who we are. Emotions are temporary and do not define us. They are a reaction to our perception of an event or a circumstance; they can even be a reaction to a mere thought or a belief. These reactions, especially when they're negative ones, can be really strong, even to the extreme of being overwhelming. Remembering that the emotions will lessen and pass is one reason to keep addressing them before they become harmful.

A helpful analogy is clouds in a blue sky. Clouds form and come and go in a huge variety of shapes, sizes, colors, and intensity. Some are wispy, light, and happy-go-lucky, and some are dark, cold, and ominous. Behind the clouds, the blue sky remains. It was there before the clouds formed, and it will be there after they have passed.

The sky is not the cloud, although something in its condition produced the cloud. In the same way, we are not our emotions. We will remain after our emotions have passed.

When we encounter emotions in others, especially strong, negative, painful ones, it can be hard to know how to react. We may want to help but not know what to do. We may start to try to help and then get drawn into the emotions ourselves. Or we may avoid the person or situation because we're unsure of the "correct" action. In my experience, daring to care is always a right action. Sitting with someone—and it may just be that, sitting—lets them know that we see their pain, that they're not alone, and that it's okay to be human. Emotions need expression. Sharing builds connections. Processing and healing depends on being heard and acknowledged.

Hearing and understanding that someone is feeling pain, however, does not mean we have to feel that same pain. If we take on the emotions of others, over time it leads to burnout, which is often called compassion fatigue. At work it can cause staff either to shut down and become desensitized in order to keep going, or to quit the field entirely. The road of compassion will ask us to go where it hurts, to share and be present in brokenness, anger, fear, and confusion. It certainly takes strength to be vulnerable and expose ourselves to this.

So how can you practice compassion and allow yourself to be a safe recipient of the message and the emotion without taking on the emotion itself? The key lies in being vigilant about two things: your greater purpose and your own emotions. First, you must remember that you are there to listen, care, acknowledge, and offer guidance if requested. When people say, "I know how you feel," it is never true. No two people have been through the same experience in the exact same way. The closest you may be able to get in sharing is to respond, reflect, and actively seek to help them find peace and direction. Stay present with them in their experience of an event and an emotion. Always know that though the emotions are not permanent and may not even be based in reality, they are perfectly real to the person having them.

Next, take inventory of your own emotions on a regular basis, especially before sitting down alongside someone who's hurting or angry. Put any unhelpful emotions you catch onto a shelf for the time being. Your attention should be focused completely on the other person. You need to be totally present for them during this time. However, remain aware of any change in your own emotions. You have to keep bringing yourself back intentionally to what is happening and why you are there.

The goal is to keep from following them into the same emotion. They are in a bad place, they may even be so emotional that it's hard to be with them. Realize that your unconditional, brave, honest attention is one of the greatest gifts that you can give to another human in these moments. When people seem the most unlovable, sometimes that's when they need our caring the most, and any connection forged will be the strongest.

It does take practice, but the more you do it, the more good you can do. Dare to care without falling in. Aim to be like the blue sky, staying there unconditionally, and show the other person that they are not their feelings. They are a blue sky too. Be sure they know that you will still be there when their feelings have run their course. You will still be connected to the person within.

Exercises for Day 23

· Keep the blue-sky vision in your mind as you encounter people and situations throughout today. Watch as clouds come and go.

· Without assuming or anticipating, simply be present with people who are angry, sad, or even happy, if you get the chance. Practice not getting angry, sad, or happy with them.

· Pay special attention to your own emotions today. Observe how your moods might go up and down, and what may have triggered the changes. It's about getting to know yourself.

Reflections

1. What emotions did I notice in myself today? When?

2. What emotionally charged situations did I run into? Was I able to stay removed and helpful to the person or people involved?

24.

Follow Through on Good Intentions

"We . . . judge ourselves by our motives—
and others by their behavior."

—STEPHEN R. COVEY

Today was my husband's birthday. I got him a card and present, and we went out to dinner. But all day long I had been intending to phone his mother in Pittsburg. Delores is ninety-six years old, and she lost her husband of sixty years—the love of her life and Kurt's father—in 2008. Now she lives alone in an apartment complex that is a NORC, a naturally occurring retirement community. She has macular degeneration and is severely visually impaired. Nevertheless, her life is full with the lifelong friends that surround her, her family, and the two sons she adores.

My intention was to call and thank her for being Kurt's mother, to share with her how grateful I am to have him in my life, and to tell her she should be proud of the incredible man that she raised and I married.

But it's 10 p.m. now and too late to call today. I can call her tomorrow, true, but it won't have exactly the same meaning. I got distracted, busy, couldn't find the number, thought maybe she'd be napping, and needed to do one more thing first.

Hopefully when I call tomorrow she'll answer; hopefully, she'll be there.

At home or at work, how many times do you think about picking up the phone to talk to a certain someone, or call to make a date for a cup of coffee or lunch? How often do you reach out to a coworker to share your break or lunchtime at work? Or think to yourself, "Hey, I should drop that person a thank you note, birthday card, condolence card, congratulations card, or just tell them something nice." And you don't.

Our best huge intentions are worth absolutely nothing compared to the smallest kind, thoughtful action. We need to let people who are important to us know that they're in our thoughts, when we are thinking of them. We never know what a huge difference we could be making in their day.

Exercises for Day 24

- People love to be thought about and cared about! Check up on someone who's been sick or is going through a difficult time. Tell them you are thinking about them. Try your best to do it with your voice or real face-to-face presence.

- Go to a coworker's office and give them a boost. Congratulate them for a job well done on a recent project or compliment them on a specific work task.

- Carve out time to say, "Hey, let's go for a quick walk." Call after a meeting and say, "You did a good job, thanks. I appreciated how you . . . ."

- Act on your intentions today. Dare to care.

Reflections

1. What intentions did I follow through on today?

2. What intentions did I have but didn't act on?

3. Why did I not act? Was it because I was distracted? Fearful? Busy? Forgot? Was it because I was procrastinating?

25.

Respond to the
Immediate Need

"Never worry about numbers. Help one person at a time
and always start with the person nearest you."

—MOTHER TERESA

Sometimes we get so caught up in the enormity of the struggles of
the world that we fail to react to the smaller need that is staring us
in the face.

It's so easy to be overwhelmed by the suffering of others and
shut ourselves off, keeping our compassion at arm's-length as a
way of lessening the pain we feel. But our true gift to others is in
what we do in the moment. These moments of opportunity don't
repeat themselves, so choose not to miss them.

Last Saturday I went to the bank to use the ATM machine.
I made a deposit and withdrew some cash. Before pulling out

of my parking spot, I was taking a minute to organize my purse when a woman appeared at my open window.

Kind of hesitantly, she said, "Excuse me, but you left a receipt in the machine." I smiled and thanked her. She smiled back and turned to leave.

I hesitated for an instant. She was middle-aged with short, blonde, messy hair. She was wearing pajama bottoms, a mismatched T-shirt, a sweatshirt, and slippers. She looked tired behind her timid smile. "How are you doing today?" I asked.

She said, "I just walked over to check our balance and hopefully get money to buy a couple of things we need." She was clearly struggling. "How much would help you?" I asked, and I met her eyes with a tiny smile. Looking at me with hope she said, "Twenty dollars."

I had just withdrawn five twenties. After considering for just a moment, I said, "Here's forty." I gave her the cash. Clearly stunned, she burst into tears. "Oh my God. Do you live here? I need your address. I can't believe this? Are you sure?" She blurted out the words. When I nodded, she continued, "I live across the street there, behind the flea market building, with my husband. He's disabled and can't work. Do you have kids in school? Our daughter goes to Sherando High. She's fifteen. What can I do for you? Oh my God."

I told her that I didn't need anything but her smile, and that because I never pull over to use the teller it seemed like we were supposed to meet. She was in need of something that I was in a position to give. After a hug and a warm smile exchanged between us, I pulled the other three twenties out of my wallet and handed them to her. "Today, you need this more than I do.

It's all I can do, and I pray it helps." She stood there dumb-founded. Blessings were exchanged, and then I put the car in reverse and backed out.

As I was getting on the interstate I thought about the inter-action and the business of charity. I thought about all the many millions of dollars that are channeled through huge organiza-tions. It's a safe, anonymous, hands-off method of helping our fellow humans, satisfying that need to be compassionate. Maybe it makes it a little easier to avoid the discomfort or unease that we feel when we actively ignore the homeless person on the street who is asking for some change or a meal, or the older person in the grocery store who has to put items back when they're being rung up, or anyone else who crosses our daily path.

At work, we may talk about caring cultures in the board room and staff meetings and then overlook a hurting employee or resi-dent, or walk past a call bell light.

We've all been there, considering whether to help or not. We can think of many reasons not to: We don't have time, we gave at the office, this person could be trying to scam me, we can't help everyone so what difference does it make.

True compassion doesn't sprout and grow at arm's-length. It happens right in front of us, in the moment and space where we are, and in the opportunities that are given to us every day. It's up to us to dare to let ourselves care enough to act.

Was I wrong in giving the money to the woman in Middle-town that Saturday? Maybe she took advantage of my kindness. One hundred dollars is not a small amount, after all, and it means a lot to me. But I think it meant the world to her. I think in this case I am happy with my choice, even if it turns out I am wrong.

To act with conscious compassion, dare to cross the distance between you and another human being with an offer of your time, hope, wisdom, humor, compassion, or even, sometimes, money.

Exercises for Day 25

· Just for today, keep your eyes wide open and recognize the needs of people around you.

· Notice when you have an impulse to reach outside of yourself to share what you have with another.

· Dare to override your discomfort. Consider whether any messages from your brain warning you not to get involved are valid.

———————— **Reflections** ————————

1. What needs did you see today?

2. Did you find yourself responding differently to opportunities to take action—or at least feeling differently about taking action?

3. Why or why not?

26.

Connect through Touch

"Studies have shown touch to be the primary language of
compassion, love and gratitude—emotions at the heart of trust
and cooperation—even more than facial expressions and voice.
Touch is the central medium in which the goodness of one
individual can spread to another."

—DACHER KELTNER

In the world of healthcare, direct care workers touch physically,
probe, and touch some more. Often the physical contact is purely
clinical. It is excruciatingly intimate, even invasive, but entirely
impersonal. This happens because of a valid need for efficiency
and adherence to standard protocols, and perhaps because of
the need for caregivers to maintain a protective and distancing
"clinical" mindset.

Is there a way that we can express more caring, respect, and compassion in our touch? Is there a way we can connect emotionally without being inappropriate? This question applies not only to direct care workers and patients but also to the employee/employer relationship.

Physical touch is one of the five basic ways that, as humans, we experience our surroundings. We touch, and we are touched, and this contributes to our understanding and interpretation of the world around us.

There is an old telephone commercial that says, "Reach out. Reach out and touch someone." It was meant to encourage people to take action and call someone who was physically apart from them. Of course, they couldn't actually *touch* the person. The simple act of the communication, though, could touch the spirit and let someone know that they were important.

Touch can be either physical or emotional. We stay connected through all sorts of technology that keeps us in touch. We can feel closer and more connected to someone who is across the country than we do with someone who is close to us physically at home or work. Connection is something that we can feel in our spirit, even over many miles. While physical touch has a powerful impact on our body, emotional connection has a profound impact on our soul. We fail to thrive without both types of touch. We are left wanting, deprived. Surviving, but not thriving, because there's something very important missing that keeps us from fully appreciating each contact with another being.

Let's consider that there is a time for clinical efficiency, and there should be moments of personal touch that acknowledge the human being behind the room or patient number. And that even when we're performing the clinical tasks, if we've fortified ourselves and our boundaries, we can perform these tasks with tenderness.

Taking time to be gentle, asking permission, telling patients what we are doing, asking if they are comfortable, asking if our touch is too rough or hands or instrument too cold will let the person know that we're aware of and care about them and their individual needs and preferences, right now. It adds an element of choice to their daily lives in a situation where they may be given so few such opportunities.

Massage in particular, even casual amateur massage, is a wonderful way to help patients relax, and rubbing lotions into elderly skin, especially feet, is helpful for healthy skin. Many elderly people have lost their life partners and can be very caring-touch deprived. Whenever possible, take the gentle approach.

In work roles such as administration, management, and non-direct care professions, touch is generally considered taboo. Inappropriate touching of coworkers or subordinates is prohibited. The definition of inappropriate is very subjective. The line between okay and not okay can be fine, and the risk of misinterpretation or even litigation so high that we basically avoid physical touch entirely. The result is that we sacrifice a tremendous tool in our communication and connection with each other in work teams, and we withhold the compassion and support that are so direly needed in the important work of health care.

We have to build trusting, respectful relationships with staff and then learn to trust ourselves before we can make responsible decisions about touch in the workplace. Depending on the person, setting, cultures, and history, we can determine where touch might be appropriate or allowed. A light touch on the shoulder or arm, or a hug, or something as simple as true eye contact with a slightly longer handshake, can have a positive impact. In my experience there are times when connecting and caring through touch is worth the risk and can demonstrate compassion in a way that words just can't. By daring to care on a physical level we're opening the door wide to deeper communication with those around us.

We're looking for ways to grow the positive impact of caring touch in our environments. We want to recognize the added value, the dimension, that touch contributes to genuine, caring interpersonal communication. Better interpersonal communication is what we're all striving for no matter where we work.

Exercises for Day 26

· Touch is a big leap. Consider—just consider—how physical touch is such an integral part of compassion. (No one is asking that you begin touching every person you encounter today!) Simply observe people around you. Often when people are talking, one will reach out and briefly touch a hand, forearm, or face. Notice couples reaching out, perhaps without even looking, for the hand of their partner.

· If you truly dare to care, be intentional about gently touching a patient just a tiny bit on their hand or arm. As you do, make soft eye contact, with your eyes slightly down, and smile warmly. Compassionate people naturally do this. Remember that we're trying to describe and define what compassion looks and feels like, so that others can practice and feel it too.

Reflections

1. What instances, if any, did I see today where touch was included as part of total communication? Did I think it enhanced the connection? Why or why not?

2. Do you believe touch is important in your work? Why or why not?

3. Describe at least one scenario where you would consider touching someone to help you show compassion to them.

27.

Question Assumptions

"If you judge people you have no time to love them."

—MOTHER TERESA

Early in my career in human resources, I was tasked with rolling out a new benefits package that included some major changes for the upcoming plan year in terms of both coverage and cost structure. We expected that the changes would be met with heavy criticism from employees. I'd prepared talking points to present the pros and cons and the rationale behind the decision. I was ready!

I kicked off the very first group meeting in a positive frame of mind, carefully explaining the choices and outlining the key elements of each level of investment. As the session progressed, I began to feel more relaxed and confident about the audience. If they weren't exactly ecstatic, they seemed willing to listen. This feeling continued as I began to wrap up and prepared to open for questions.

Then I noticed a stern-looking man seated along the back wall. His arms were solidly crossed, and he was steadily shaking his head back and forth. He became all that I could see. In my mind, his disapproval clouded the room.

My mood dropped, my confidence plummeted, and my attitude toward the entire group became defensive, frustrated, and disappointed. The meeting that I thought was going so well suddenly could not be over soon enough. I'm sure that my insecurity tainted the rest of the gathering. Later, I was debriefing with my supervisor, and I shared about the man in the back row. Imagine my surprise when she said, "Oh, that's Tom. He's in the early stages of Parkinson's disease. It affects his nervous system so that he has tremors and head shakes."

I've never forgotten Tom, that incident, or the lesson it taught me. I've learned to recognize when I'm making assumptions based on what may be false evidence. I have learned to adjust my actions accordingly. If I do make assumptions, I have learned to try to assume the best rather than the worst.

Intentional compassion and understanding of others requires an open heart and the absence of judgment and assumptions. This means being more mindful and looking beyond what seems obvious. It means being aware of the occasions when we're letting preconceived notions affect our interpretation, our emotions, and thus our response to people and situations.

These notions might well be based on erroneous information:

- Outward appearances, such as the physical behavior of the man in my story, that shape our choice of action

- Subtle, misinterpreted signals, like a shared smile or whisper, or abruptly ended conversation that causes us to believe someone is talking about us and affects how we respond to them

- Assumptions about another person, such as: "They're strong, they don't need my help," that cause us to neglect someone who is uncomfortable asking for assistance

- Our negative belief about the future, such as "This meeting is going to go badly," which causes us to approach events with low expectations

- Or a poor judgment that's based on past experience, which we accept as equally true for this new person or day; for example, if we think a patient is always grumpy, we put up protective barriers and don't share the best we have to give

The best first step is to proactively guard against a false assumption by looking at where a belief is rooted. Clear out the unreal and replace it with the willingness to move forward with a clean slate. Approach every person and every encounter in a neutral, receptive way. This demands bravery, a sense of curiosity and exploration, and a daring-to-care attitude—all vital characteristics of the compassionate leader.

Be vigilant about any new assumptions you make. It takes time and practice, but it will become a habit. Your reward will be a more realistic view of the people and the world around you.

Exercises for Day 27

- Focus today on identifying where false assumptions are *hurting* you.

- Reflect on a past situation where you assumed the worst about an outcome or a person (like I did), and you were wrong.

- Next, remind yourself of a time when you falsely believed the *best* of someone, you were wrong, and you wish that you had looked more honestly and openly at the facts. Guarding against assumptions works both ways; you must approach today with an open, receptive mind if you want to see clearly.

—————————— **Reflections** ——————————

1. What do I think about assumptions? Are they important? Did I find myself assuming something today that I shouldn't have? If so, what was it?

2. How can I avoid assumptions that hurt me? What will I do differently tomorrow?

3. How do assumptions affect my ability to be compassionate?

28.

First, Practice
Self-Compassion

"In the event of a sudden loss of cabin pressure, place an oxygen mask
on yourself before assisting children or other passengers."

—STANDARD AIRLINE SAFETY INSTRUCTIONS

It's a fact! We can't care for others for any extended period of time
if we don't put ourselves first. It may seem selfish, but the human
soul needs genuine, healthy self-compassion in order to gift compassion to those around us.

Burnout is a significant and growing concern among healthcare workers, whether they are on the front line as nurses or aides
or in support occupations such as human resources, administration, or social services. People become burned out when they
ignore their boundaries and give too much; this results in feeling
they've been taken advantage of, or feeling completely exhausted.

Healthcare attracts caring souls, but some people allow themselves to be used well beyond their reserves of compassion or empathy. Burnout may cause them to leave the organization, or worse, the healthcare field, believing that it is the industry or company that's at fault. In the very worst-case scenario, they stay despite the burnout, completely disconnected from the environment and functioning in survival mode.

We need to educate staff about self-compassion in our workplaces and provide and support outlets to achieve it. Self-care must be a recurring agenda item on staff meeting agendas. We need to give staff space and time to share and realize they are not alone. As leaders, we need to be openly compassionate with our staff, to be vulnerable and approachable so that they can work through the emotions of this very demanding and vital work that we do.

From my years in healthcare, I have confidence in the compassionate qualities of the majority of the people on the front line. As leaders, we can truly support them, beyond teaching and investing in self-care programs, by acting as buffers for stressors from "higher-ups" that affect them in their daily work. Another way is to demonstrate a healthy approach to work-life balance by doing things as simple as taking breaks and lunches, taking days off, and limiting extended work hours. Give staff a sounding board for their issues. If we model self-care behaviors as leaders, staff will see that's it's good for them to practice those behaviors too.

All of this is a deep subject and a tall order. There is so much work and education to be done, and the field is only now waking up to the dire urgency of the need.

For now, act as your own best friend. It is not weak to care for yourself, it is your responsibility. Pay attention to what it is you need, and when those needs aren't being met. Honor the requirement for care and attention to yourself because it is absolutely necessary in order to continue this work that you are called to do.

Be the change. Take care of yourself so you can take care of others. You and those you serve will be better for it.

Exercises for Day 28

- Today, find some good information on self-care or stress management for medical professionals online or in a magazine or book. Add a brief discussion of the information to the agenda for your next staff meeting so you can introduce the subject.

- Carve out quiet time. You require a bit of stillness if you're going to be able to offer a healing compassionate touch in your encounters today. Try, no matter how busy or active your day. Leaders help make compassion happen!

---------------------------- **Reflections** ----------------------------

1. My quiet moments today were . . .

2. I knew the quiet moments helped me when . . .

3. Starting tomorrow, here are three things I'm going to do to take better care of my work self:

Conclusion

Imagine for just a moment that you have discovered an incredible medicine, something that can cure a major disease or alleviate the suffering of people who are in pain. It's ready to go; all you need is the delivery method. Let's imagine that the incredible, healing "medicine" is compassion. Something we all innately possess, we just have to know how to "do" it.

It seems like every day we're offered a new remedy, a new strategy or system, or a new technology designed to increase our personal and professional effectiveness and ease the "pains" of our work and its challenges, the "ills of society."

The goal of these remedies is to achieve a higher-quality outcome and make our lives easier. The questions are: What's working and what's not? Why? What, if any, results are lasting, and can we build on them? It seems we just continue to work harder with less, against higher demands. The resources, human and otherwise, are stretched and sometimes they fail. But always we press ahead.

There is an irony in that generally we seek to overcome these challenges with one-size-fits-all people solutions, when people are fundamentally and beautifully diverse. A unique identifier of humans, the great equalizer, is that we all need to give and receive compassion. Compassion is different for each person and situation, yet it is always compassion.

What began for me as a theory, which then became a belief, and is now a conviction is that the strategy, or size, that fits the one *and* the all is compassion.

Maya Angelou said, "I've learned that people will forget what you said, people will forget what you did, but people will never forget how you made them feel."

How are you making people feel? Where are you as leaders and care providers taking your organizations? Let's replace the word *organizations* with the word *stakeholders*—the employees, residents, patients, their families, your communities, your corporate business partners.

Communication is frequently cited as the biggest single threat to organizational effectiveness. So the potential success of any organization is limited only by the strength and core competencies of its leaders.

These are the conclusions I want you to reach about compassion:

Compassion is a universal answer to the challenges facing not only healthcare but also academia, the business world, and society in all its beautiful manifestations.

Compassion transcends stereotyping, labeling, profiling, bias, judgment, opinions, language, and culture. Compassion is the ultimate in person-centered care.

Compassion is timeless. It is a fundamental human need and

drive. It will never go out of style. It will never be the wrong time or circumstance to show compassion.

Compassion has to be a fundamentally understood and agreed-upon value of any caring culture. It must start at the top of any existing hierarchy and permeate every layer of the group.

Compassion has different definitions. It is more helpful to study what it looks like in action and practice those behaviors, so we can be more intentionally thoughtful in our interactions with others.

Compassion is free yet priceless.

If you accept these conclusions and recognize compassion for what it is, a lasting cornerstone rather than a program or "flavor of the month," then I applaud you.

Are there obstacles to growing the seeds of compassion in our workplaces and our lives? Yes. We've examined many of them in this book. Yet we can always do better, learning about ourselves and what makes us do what we do. The principles laid out here—Listen, Engage, Act, and Dare to Care (LEAD)—are a pathway that gives us a starting point as well as a compass to guide us on our travels. It's a destination at which we'll never "arrive"; we'll simply continue on a journey of exploring the truth of who we are as humans, being.

Albert Einstein said, "I have deep faith that the principle of the universe will be beautiful and simple." Compassion is this beautiful and simple principle I believe, in relation to humanity.

As a leader, and a giver of care, what do you believe? What will be the legacy that you leave with those you touch? Let it be a journey of human exploration that begins and ends with compassion.

Next Steps:
The Compassion Component

There are three levels of commitment that will instill a deeper understanding of compassion in your organization. Consider how you could take action to "deliver" the compassion component.

Awareness Level:

Goal = Highlighting understanding compassion and encouraging further learning among staff.

- Orient senior leaders to compassion.

- Host an informational all-staff meeting with a guest speaker to introduce compassion.

- Encourage department heads to explore and discuss compassion in group meetings and one-on-ones.

- Use *28 Ways of Compassion* as appropriate to promote further study of compassion and its effects in the workplace.

- Keep the discussion alive.

Initiative Level:

Goal = Adopt *28 Ways of Compassion* as a semiformal initiative at the organizational level

- Secure commitments from board members and senior leaders to create a compassionate organization.
- Schedule a kick-off All-Staff meeting.
- Schedule a series of at least four half-day in-service trainings for current staff with a custom curriculum coordinated through The Compassion Component.
- Create or adapt a module for use in the orientation of new employees (including new manager training) as well as new residents. (Optional: videotape for alternate use.)
- Develop methods for celebrating compassion moments.

Champion Level:

Description = Commit to hardwiring compassion into the organization and to being a pilot project for research on the ROI of compassionate ways.

- Before any formal communication or training on compassion begins,
  - Champions will commit to project objectives, plan, measurement intervals, and timelines.

- Champions will work with researchers to identify 5 to 7 measurable performance indicators (PIs) at their site or organization (ex: call bell usage). Optimally these PIs will reflect areas where there is a current need for improvement or specific concerns.

- Pre- and post-training measurements will be taken.

- Champions agree to the publication of results in a future book (anonymously if desired). The book is tentatively titled *Compassion in Healthcare: From Boardroom to Bedside.* It will be a detailed study including data, stories, and lessons learned from participating groups. Project results may also be shared at health care and customer care conferences.

- Champions will complete the actions listed under the Initiative Level.

Champions will earn the designation of "Compassion Champions" (or some similar title), and all staff will receive a lapel pin that signifies compassion.

About the Author

Denise D. Borgoyn has over 35 years of experience in the health and human services fields. "Dee's" career has spanned high-level human resources management and leadership in government, not-for-profit, and Fortune 500 companies. She is a sought-after expert, speaker, and consultant in health care, diversity, specifically disability and aging issues, and workforce and customer service strategies.

She is committed to people and facing challenges, and has been a pioneer all her life in advocating for people, and creating

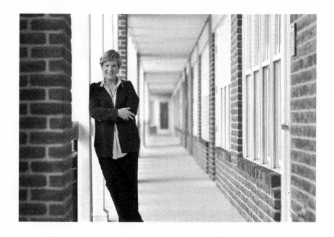

solutions; active in the development of the Americans With Disabilities Act, founder of Nevada's "Jobs for the Handicapped" in 1982, a grant-funded program that is still in operation, serving returning veterans after the Vietnam War, acting as a Wounded Warrior Mentor for today's returning soldiers, coaching disabled children and adults (as she is disabled from birth herself), pushing for cancer research as the mother of a childhood cancer survivor, and now, championing the study and practice of compassion in healthcare.

Dee is an expert in leadership development and coaching, workforce strategies, person-centered health care, and diversity and inclusion for persons with disabilities. The bulk of her experience has been in health care arenas, focusing on people processes and systems as they relate to gerontology, aging services, and long-term care. Dee has worked with medium and large retirement communities, community agencies, home health, hospice, hospitals, and free-standing clinic systems. She built an especially strong customer service skillset while a senior leader for Spiegel's telecommunications service centers, leveraging those skills by applying them to direct care of healthcare customers.

Dee holds a B.S. in Special Education with a Psychology minor from the University of Nevada, Reno. She is an active member of the Washington, D.C., chapter of the National Speakers Association, a Senior Certified Professional in Human Resources (SHRM-SCP), a licensed Nursing Home Administrator in the Commonwealth of Virginia, a past state President and Regional Representative for The American Society for HealthCare Human

Resources Administration (American Hospital Association). She was named Outstanding Young Woman by the Nevada attorney general.

She lives on a small historic farm in Virginia at the top of the Shenandoah Valley, with her husband Kurt and a menagerie of mini-goats, angora bunnies, horses, dogs and assorted chickens.

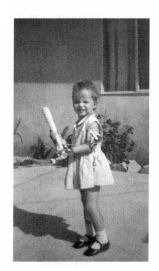

Contacting Dee

Dee is available to speak to your organization, group, or conference globally about compassion and caring work cultures. Other services include consulting and strategic work sessions, as well as customized programming.

Your questions and comments are welcomed, along with any stories you would like to share with us about compassion in health care.

To arrange for her to address your organization or other group, please visit her website at www.deeborgoyn.com or email her at dee@deeborgoyn.com.